FASCIA

What It Is and Why It Matters

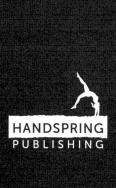

HANDSPRING
PUBLISHING

David Lesondak

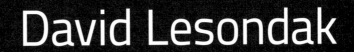

What It Is and Why It Matters

Forewords
Thomas W. Myers
Robert Schleip
Carla Stecco

Afterwords
Thomas W. Findley
Sasha Chaitow

SECOND EDITION

First published in Great Britain in 2017 by
Handspring Publishing
This second edition published in 2023 by
Handspring Publishing, an imprint of Jessica Kingsley Publishers
An imprint of Hodder & Stoughton Ltd
An Hachette UK Company

1

A CIP catalogue record for this title is available from the British Library and the Library of Congress

ISBN 978 1 91342 631 6
eISBN 978 1 83997 598 1

Printed and bound in Great Britain by Bell and Bain Limited

Jessica Kingsley Publishers' policy is to use papers that are natural, renewable and recyclable products and made from wood grown in sustainable forests. The logging and manufacturing processes are expected to conform to the environmental regulations of the country of origin.

Handspring Publishing
Carmelite House
50 Victoria Embankment
London EC4Y 0DZ

www.handspringpublishing.com

CONTENTS

CONTENTS *continued*

ABOUT THE AUTHOR

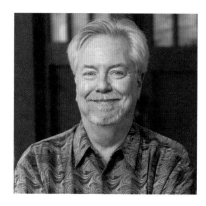

David Lesondak BCSI, ATSI, FST, FFT, VMT is an Allied Health Member in the Department of Family and Community Medicine at the University of Pittsburgh Medical Center (UPMC). He serves as the Senior Structural Integrator and Fascia Specialist at UPMC's Center for Integrative Medicine. He has been a clinical bodyworker for over 30 years. He is a Board Certified Structural Integrator, Frederick Stretch Therapist Level 2, Fascial Fitness Trainer, and Visceral Manipulator via the Barral Institute.

David is the author of the international best seller *Fascia: What it is and why it matters*. His follow-up book *Fascia, Function, and Medical Applications* was nominated for a 2021 British Medical Association award. He has also contributed chapters to the 2nd edition of *Fascia: The Tensional Network of the Human Body* and the 2nd edition of *Metabolic Therapies In Orthopedics*. He has also contributed to the 4th edition of Joe Muscolino's *Kinesiology*.

David sits on the Executive Committee of the International Consortium on Manual Therapies.

A passionate and engaging speaker of all things fascia, David has been an invited speaker and workshop facilitator to such diverse groups as the National Institutes of Health (NIH) Workshop on Myofascial Pain, the Academic Consortium of Integrative Medicine, the Performance, Health, and Wellness Staff for the LA Clippers, both the British and Australian Fascia Symposiums, the World Fascia Congress, the Anatomy Trains Masterclass Series, the University of Arizona College of Medicine, and many others.

He hosts the podcast BodyTalk with David Lesondak.

Before entering the healthcare field in 1991, David's various career incarnations were in television, advertising, the funeral arts, and over a decade-long stint as a DJ on WYEP-FM in Pittsburgh. He maintains an avid interest in music and songwriting.

His website is www.davidlesondak.com.

DEDICATION

In Memoriam

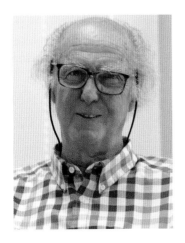

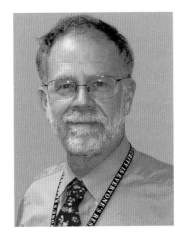

Leon Chaitow (1937–2018)

Tom Findley (1949–2021)

The second edition of this book is dedicated to the memory of
Leon Chaitow and Tom Findley who furthered the acceptance of manual
therapy in the realm of medicine, were rigorous about their science,
and understood the importance of paying it forward.

FOREWORD by Thomas W. Myers

Eric McLuhan, the son of the great media expert Marshall McLuhan, taught me to speed read in 1970 – a talent I have been grateful for ever since. But his opening line was: Would you rather spend 45 minutes reading a summary of the book or in conversation with the author? Everyone answers "In conversation with the author."

I can personally assure you that David Lesondak is a brilliant and engaging conversationalist. This book is exactly like having a talk with him – his personal whimsical style and humor shine through, the wide variety of his interests are in evidence at every turn. David has a way of explaining complex ideas in understandable terms without dulling the scientific edge or cheapening the argument.

You can take this book home with you and enjoy it all at once as a great big meal, or snack on it in pieces – either way you will be assured of tasty and nutritious food for your mind. It has the additional benefit of being fresh – the scientific information on fascia is accurate and up to date.

It has been my pleasure to know David for over a decade as a student, colleague, and teacher, and this book is an absolutely quintessential expression of his dedication to accuracy, his panoramic scope, and his infectious enthusiasm for the living fabric of the body.

Tom Myers

Clarks Cove, Maine

June 2017

FOREWORD by Robert Schleip

When I invited David to use his video skills to document the first Fascia Summer School in 2010 I had no idea what I was in for. Neither, I think, did he.

Though we had met several years previously, it was over the ensuing seven years that every time I turned around at a major conference David was there; behind his cameras, capturing all the moments, and later meticulously editing the lectures for maximum clarity.

I came to realize there was a very keen mind behind that camera, putting theories and ideas together in some very unique ways over the many conversations and teaching opportunities that we have shared. This was very apparent in his many intelligent questions, with which he interspersed his frequent personal interviews with our keynote presenters, and also in his own active input in the many discussions that surround an effective scientific meeting. In fact, I was so much impressed by David's personal knowledge of the fascia research field and his own ideas in this area that we gave him the opportunity to lecture himself at our bi-annual Fascia Research Summer School at Ulm University. However, I was not prepared for the mastery and brilliance with which he filled that slot and impressed even me.

So too, I suspect, he will surprise you as you read his book. Whether you are new to the wonderful world of fascia or an old-timer like myself, you will find ideas, images, and impeccably explained science, written in a way that is both illuminating and memorably entertaining. At the same time, this book will serve as a valuable reference with which to dive deeper into study as you see fit.

This is a true masterpiece. It takes the reader on an entertaining journey into "fascia land" from both a lay person's and a clinician's perspective. I will definitely ask David for permission to use some of his elegant and impressive illustrations, concepts, and creative analogies in my own teaching and writing in the future. We will also make sure David is no longer solely "behind the cameras" at our international events but in front of them as well. What he has to share it truly too good to miss.

Perhaps because of my own professional journey, one of my favorite things is watching a clinician make the journey from "therapy land" into "science land." When I first met David, I thought he might be one of those clinicians. But never did I expect that ten years later I would be reading a book like this.

I cannot wait to see what he does in the next ten years. I will be first in line.

Robert Schleip

Munich, Germany

June 2017

FOREWORD by Carla Stecco

To write the foreword of a book is always an honor, above all when it is about a topic of particular importance to me, as fascia is.

I know David from many years of going to fascia symposia and "summer schools" at the University of Ulm, Leipzig, and other universities and locations. It was during discussions at those events that I noticed his tremendous enthusiasm for fascia and his great capacity to communicate the latest scientific discoveries in simple and accurate ways.

I think this book is the perfect expression of David's thoughts.

In this book the reader will find, written in a simple but comprehensive way, everything there is to know about fascia: the definition, the macroscopic and microscopic anatomy, the biomechanics with the various models, the history, the clinical applications, the diagnostic tools, everything. All the chapters are rich in figures and references, and always maintain a high scientific level.

David moves well between the problems related to the definition of fascia and the various biomechanical models, presenting both specific anatomical continuities and more global visions of fascia. He also dedicates many pages to the history of fascial discoveries, and I feel honored that he included me in this part.

Another interesting and new area is related to the nervous system and considers not only fascial innervation but also the relationship with the brain. The other chapters are more focused on clinical applications and diagnostic tools to detect and evaluate fascial alterations.

The book is clear, concise, and very readable.

I recommend it to everyone who is interested in understanding all of the main concepts of fascia.

Carla Stecco

Professor of Human Anatomy and Movement Science

University of Padua

Padua, Italy

May 2022

PREFACE

"I should write a book one day" – how many of us think that? Most of us, I'll wager – myself included.

Many people tell me what an accomplishment it is that I have actually done just that. Honestly, it does not feel that way from the inside.

It was a thorough pleasure. Of course there were moments...moments where it felt as if what I wanted to say was somehow bigger than my brain could contain. And then those moments had to be funneled through my brain and mouth and down into finger words. Writing is a mechanical process. It is also a cranial, thinking process. It is "both/and" – somewhat like fascia.

So as I think about how this book came to be I keep coming back to one specific thing, and three people that I would like to blame.

What was the specific thing? I was there.

My quest to find more reliable outcomes for my patients, those who entrusted me with being the custodian and wayfinder for the way out of their chronic pain, led me to the world of fascia – and that world turned out to be a whole inner universe.

I had the good fortune to be there as the science behind the practical, clinical results was crystallizing and being born. We were all taking our first steps as researchers and clinicians and were just keeping our heads above water. But delightfully so.

Sometimes the science offered tantalizing answers, and just as often led to even more tantalizing connections and questions. But, by and large, we were all buoyed by the idea that *we were on to something*, and that something was special. Something so special yet so ubiquitous as

to be overlooked because it seemed as common as water is to fish and air is to mammals. Fascia. Connective tissue.

And I was there, duly documenting the conferences since 2007, editing the videos, exploring the techniques, and extrapolating from the potential clinical applications of science to create, often in the moment, new approaches to improve and accelerate the outcomes for my patients.

It is my absolute joy to bring you the results of my having been there in this book.

Now the blame.

I blame my fifth-grade science teacher who told me we only use 10 per cent of our brain. This made no sense to me at all back then, and I resolved in that moment that I would use more than 10 per cent, that I would use as much of my brain as possible. I mean, why else is it there? (See Chapter 5 for more on that.)

Next I blame my tailor in the second grade. It was my first communion and I was getting my pants hemmed for this special occasion. As the tailor was taking measurements and pinning up the hems he made the comment that one of my legs was longer than the other. This comment deeply disturbed me. I thought something had to be wrong with me and I told him so. "Don't worry," he said casually. "It's normal. Everyone's like that."

This also made no sense to me. And it haunted me. How could *that* be *normal*? So, the answers to my puzzlement about that are strewn across Chapters 1, 2, 3, and 7.

And finally I need to blame my parents. Because that's what we do.

My father worked in the steel mills of Pittsburgh. He was a riveter and he worked hard — very hard — and often with a rivet gun in each hand to get the job done on time. He took pride in the segments of bridges he put together and would often point them out to me on Sunday drives. He was also a bookie (but that's an entirely different book).

Dad would come home from a hard day at the mills and I would see my mother dab alcohol onto cotton balls and swab his back to get the grit and dirt out. She was also, to a degree, massaging the tissues and providing a different kind of stimulus to his nervous system. Not that I knew any of that at the time. My mother just told me she was "alcoholing his back." Nonetheless, it made him feel better, and I began to associate touch with well-being.

My mother employed similar techniques with me when I was restless and could not sleep, which was often, but without the alcohol. She would often sing to me as she did so and most often it was this:

> *Oh, the foot bone's connected to the ankle bone,*
> *The ankle bone's connected to the leg bone,*
> *The leg bone's connected to the thigh bone,*
> *The thigh bone's connected to the hip bone...*

and so on all the way up my body. I never tired of our ritual, and I now wonder if sometimes I pretended to be restless because I enjoyed it so much.

So at an early age I understood that it is all connected. Now, at a much later age, let me show you how.

Our journey begins on the next page...

David Lesondak

Pittsburgh, PA, USA

May 2022

ACKNOWLEDGMENTS

Jean-Claude Guimberteau told me that writing a book is always a personal adventure, "an achievement of personal experiences and a desire to share." Very true, and *merci beaucoup, Jean-Claude, pour votre générosité.*

What is even truer is that none of these experiences and adventures would ever have happened without a web of incredible people who helped me along the way.

Firstly, thank you to every person, patient, or client who has been on my treatment table. Your desire to understand what was going on with your body fueled my own curiosity for deeper insights. The same goes to every student it has been my privilege to teach. Your questions inspired me to search for clearer understanding.

Thanks to Kerma Stanton and Earl Timberlake, my first bodywork teachers, and to all the great yoga teachers I have been privileged to study with: "Black Belt" Kate (in 1985), Joyce Tillotson, Donna Dyer, Kim Phillips, Monique Richards, Max Strom, and Kendell Romanelli. You have done this body good and given me more than you know.

Thanks to Brenda Weisner for making school bearable and being a great cadaver buddy, and to Philip Newstead for being a great study buddy. Thanks also to Kana Moll for her grace, playfulness, and amazing way with words.

Thank you to Gary Vlachos for giving me my first job, Betty Kargocos for taking me seriously and referring so many people to my practice (and giving me a copy of *Anatomy Trains!*), and Christine Troples for introducing me to structural integration. *Muchos, muchos gracias* to Phil Harris for being a partner in crime for so many years, and being a truly good and forgiving friend.

Richard Finn, gentleman, scholar, and master teacher – thank you for taking me in and giving me regular opportunities to speak the language of anatomy. I became fluent because of your kindness. And thank you to Carol Finn, for always making me laugh and always having brilliantly annoying questions. *Mucho amor.*

Much love and gratitude goes to Simone Lindner for always having my back. Thanks to Carrie Gaynor for encouraging my storytelling in our early days of teaching together. Thanks to Jenny Otto for holding ladders, cameras, and being a great video assistant during some crucial adventures.

Kudos to the incredible team at UPMC Center for Integrative Medicine. Thank you for all the support, especially in 2016 when I was writing this, and for opening the door to the wider world of integrative medicine, which feels like home to me. Likewise, Dr. Bern Bernacke – thank you for all the mentoring. Without your guidance and insistence that I publish, this book might not exist. To Drs. Gary Chimes, Neilly Buckalew, and Eric Helm – it has been absolute pleasure to collaborate with you over the years.

To George Kousaleos: Pós boró poté na sas epistrépso gia tis pollés, pollés kalosýni sas kai vathiá filía?

Muchas gracias to Bibiana Badenes for bringing me to beautiful Benicassim. I think I got the best part of that deal.

Vielen Dank to Werner Klingler for your warmth and caring. Thanks to Ann and Chris Frederick for many years of friendship and that fateful train ride in Germany. Thank you to Gary Carter, my brother in the UK, Lauri Nemetz, for always being

ACKNOWLEDGMENTS *continued*

willing to lend a hand, and Rachelle Clauson, for your energy, enthusiasm, and effectiveness.

Thanks to PJ O'Clair for being a) awesome, b) awesome, and c) awesome. I hope we have more adventures together. You're the best!

Thank you to my sister Leslie for all the love, support, and enthusiasm for my chosen vocation. And especially for taking dictation and helping organize the outline that became this book.

Thanks to the team at Handspring Publishing: Andrew, for the fateful invitation; Sarena, for your patience and faith; Sally, for your scrupulous attention to detail; Mary, Hilary, Martin, Morven, and Bruce, for the utmost pleasant professionalism – every first-time author should have it so good.

To the new team at Jessica Kingsley, I'm just getting to know all of you, but it feels like the beginning of a beautiful friendship.

Thanks to Heidi Patterson, aka Chanandler Bung, research librarian extraordinaire, and a good friend. You are the living embodiment of what Neil Gaiman meant when he said: "Google can bring you back, you know, a 100,000 answers. A librarian can bring you back the right one."

And thank you, Google, for being there at 2 am, when I could not call Heidi. She really doesn't appreciate that sort of thing.

Unbelievable gratitude to my life partner Coletta Perry who has been teaching me about "both/and" for over 28 years. She is also the one who declared: "If you're going to write a book about fascia you have to say what it is and why it matters."

Finally, thank you to Tom Myers for showing me the path, Robert Schleip for taking me to the mountain, and Tom Findley for teaching me how to ski down it.

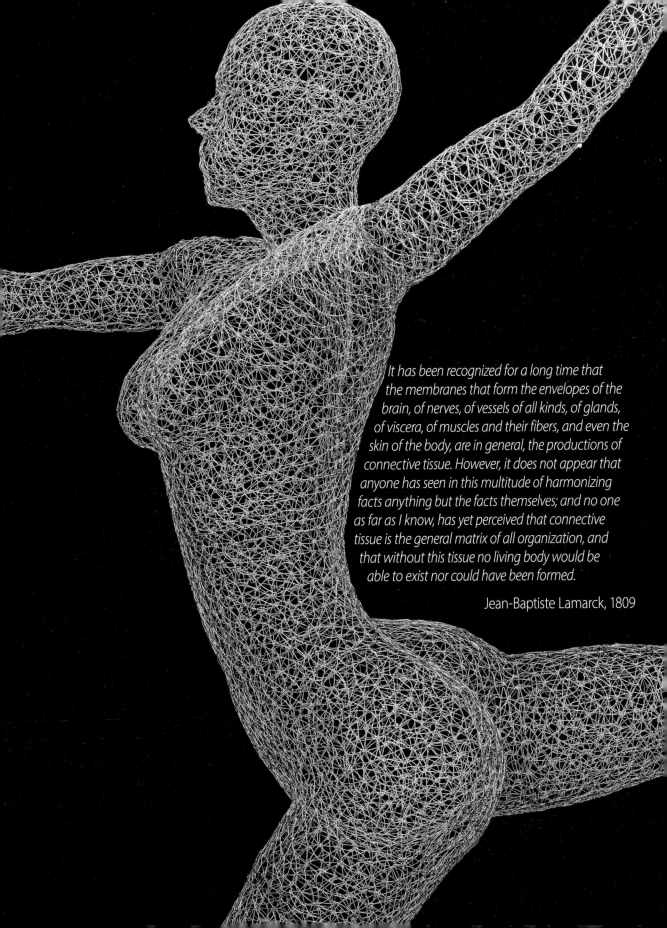

It has been recognized for a long time that the membranes that form the envelopes of the brain, of nerves, of vessels of all kinds, of glands, of viscera, of muscles and their fibers, and even the skin of the body, are in general, the productions of connective tissue. However, it does not appear that anyone has seen in this multitude of harmonizing facts anything but the facts themselves; and no one as far as I know, has yet perceived that connective tissue is the general matrix of all organization, and that without this tissue no living body would be able to exist nor could have been formed.

Jean-Baptiste Lamarck, 1809

Fascia: The Living Tissue and System

Experience teaches that it takes years or decades for new fundamental insights in medicine to become common knowledge among doctors.

Additionally, any body of knowledge that reveals linear (or) causal relationships is more easily understood and categorized than those that reveal relationships that are multidimensional.

—Gisela Draczynski

A not-so-simple definition of fascia

On September 17, 2015, the Nomenclature Committee of the Fascia Research Congress came to consensus on the anatomical definition of fascia. This was at the request of the IFAA – the International Federation of Associations of Anatomists. This was a big deal.

The IFAA is responsible for maintaining the *Terminologia Anatomica*, which sets the international standard for terminology in human anatomy. While that might seem overly obvious, there was a time when the 5,000 structures in the body were referred to by approximately 50,000 different terms (Adstrum 2014). In this capacity the IFAA performs a vital function. Given that the term "fascia" can and has been used rather broadly, the IFAA recognized the need for a new standard definition of fascia and went to the world experts in the field.

So, on September 18, 2015, at the Fourth International Fascia Research Congress, Carla Stecco MD presented the new, medical definition of fascia to the 700 plus attendees: "Fascia," she declared, "is a sheath, a sheet, or any number of other dissectible aggregations of connective tissue that forms beneath the skin to attach, enclose, and separate muscles and other internal organs" (Stecco C. 2015).

To some this was a letdown, to some it was a great moment, and to others it actually felt controversial. In a world where consensus is so hard to come by, why wasn't this breakthrough being unanimously celebrated?

Perhaps it is because in 2007 at the First International Fascia Research Congress, Robert Schleip and Thomas Findley defined fascia as follows:

Fascia is the soft tissue component of the connective tissue system that permeates the human body, forming a whole-body continuous three-dimensional matrix of structural support. It interpenetrates and surrounds all organs, muscles, bones, and nerve fibers, creating a unique environment for body systems functioning. **The scope of our definition** [my emphasis] *and interest in fascia extends to all fibrous connective tissues including aponeurosis, ligaments, tendons, retinacula, joint capsules, organ and vessel tunics...* (Findley & Schleip 2007)

Chapter One

Now you know why some attendees were disappointed. How could such an integral tissue – some call fascia the "the organ of form" (Varela & Frenk 1987, Garfin et al. 1981) – be limited by such a narrow definition?

If one's interest in fascia is coming from a purely histological, microscopic, or morphological tissue-and-structure perspective then it makes sense to have a very narrow definition. However, if one's interest is more functional or sensory and if one is curious about the way fascia behaves, then a much broader definition is necessary. Fascia is both a tissue and a system, and as such it has certain properties and functions that were not even hinted at in the new definition for the IFAA.

The good news for those underwhelmed and frustrated by the 2015 announcement (so, all of us really) is that a second *functional* definition of the fascial system has been forthcoming, it is even better than the 2007 definition and it only took four additional years to arrive at that consensus.

The fascial system consists of the three-dimensional continuum of soft, collagen containing, loose and dense fibrous connective tissues that permeate the body.

It incorporates elements such as adipose tissue, adventitiae and neurovascular sheaths, aponeuroses, deep and superficial fasciae, epineurium, joint capsules, ligaments, membranes, meninges, myofascial expansions, periostea, retinacula, septa, tendons, visceral fasciae, and all the intramuscular and intermuscular connective tissues including endomysium/ perimysium/epimysium.

The fascial system surrounds, interweaves between, and interpenetrates all organs, muscles, bones, and nerve fibers, endowing the body with structure, and providing an environment that enables all body systems to operate in an integrated manner. (Schleip et al. 2019)

It all sounds more than a bit like Obi-Wan Kenobi or Yoda describing the Force. Back in our galaxy it also resonates, for me anyway, with recent revelations about the mycelial network – a vast interconnected underground network among fungi, and other flora (Fricker et al. 2021). Noted for its plastic, adaptable qualities and how molecular events can affect the whole network at scale – the parallels are fascinating. But we're talking about humans here, not mushrooms, so let us reorient and begin to comprehend fascia – the most universal, and perhaps most misunderstood, tissue in the body.

Fascia 101

Anatomy and rehabilitation professor Andry Vleeming once said: "Fascia is your soft skeleton" (Vleeming 2011). That's a great way to think about fascia in relation to the hard skeleton of your bones. Unlike your bones, however, the most important thing to keep foremost in mind, at all times, is that your fascial net is one continuous structure throughout the body.

I will certainly use specific terminologies and clearly identified structures (i.e., the mesentery, the deltoid, etc.) but I will do so topographically, so we know where we are on the map. As far as the body is concerned, the fascia is all one – one complex, holistic, self-regulating organ/tissue/system. It is capable of being dissected out in pieces to study, obviously, but it is no less a singular unit in nature than the organ/tissue/system known as the skin. How many pieces or parts does the skin have? It is the same with the fascia.

The ubiquity of fascia – it is literally everywhere in the body–has made it very difficult to image in any useful way. Recent innovations in ultrasound and computer-assisted imaging, up to and including 3D printing, however, point to a moment in the not-too-distant future when we may have a fully realized image of the fascial net. And in Chapter 3, we will cover a very recent, highly complicated (but much more lower tech by comparison), twenty-first century attempt to envision the reality of the fascial body in all of its complicated splendor.

The "everywhereness" of fascia also implies that, indeed, *it is all connected*, and thus is "connective tissue," which is a term often used interchangeably with "fascia." There is also the quite evocative German word for connective tissue *bindgewebe*, which makes me think of "binding web," and from this we get to "fascial web." Please note that we will be using the terms "fascial net," "fascial web," and "fascial system" interchangeably to prevent jargon fatigue.

So, imagine a silvery-white material (Figure 1.1), flexible and sturdy in equal measure – a substance that surrounds and penetrates every muscle, coats every bone, covers every organ, and envelops every nerve. Fascia keeps everything separate yet interconnected at the same time. It is a tissue that up until recently was thought to be inert and lifeless (Schleip 2005,

Schleip et al. 2006). Welcome to the fascia and the fascial web.

So now that we have the unity of fascia clearly in our minds, let's do what humans love to do: take it apart to see how it all works! Don't worry – we will also be putting it back together and hopefully there will be no parts left over when we're done.

There have been many attempts to categorize fascia in the broader sense. One common categorization is to make the fascia of the limbs appendicular and distinct from the fascia of the back and torso. Another well-meaning attempt (Kumka & Bonar 2012) suggested organizing fascia into four functional categories: linking, fascicular, compression, and separating. As interesting as that idea is, it quickly gets so complicated that you might want to turn around and head back when we have only just begun our journey.

So, to keep things relatable we will make four distinctions for fascia, based on location.

Superficial fascia

The superficial layer is often described as a fibrous layer of loose connective tissue. Loose because there is not a strong, regular pattern to its organization (Figure 1.2). This layer is also often described as "areolar," which can be confusing

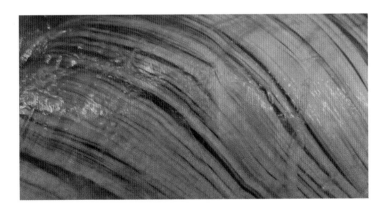

Figure 1.1
Close-up of the fascia surrounding a muscle in an unembalmed cadaver.
Photo by author. Reproduced with kind permission from Thomas W. Myers.

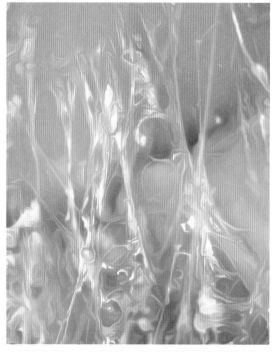

Figure 1.2
High in lubricating glycosaminoglycans like hyaluronan, loose connective tissue can be found wherever sliding, gliding, and cushioning is required. Collagen fibers can be found within its watery matrix, but the organization is loose and highly adaptable to its surroundings.
Photo by Nicole Trombley and Rachelle Clauson. Courtesy of AnatomySCAPES.com.

until one realizes that "areolar" comes from the Latin "area," meaning "open place." Superficial fascia is also called pannicular fascia, from the medical term panniculus, which comes from the Latin "pannus" meaning a piece of cloth. It is also referred to as the "hypodermis" by the *Nomina Anatomica*, also adding another impediment to clarity and interdisciplinary understanding.

Superficial fascia is the fascial membrane directly underneath a slightly more superficial layer of adipose tissue under the skin (Figure 1.3). It is fibrous yet highly elastic (about 13 per cent of the fibers are elastic) and has a variable fat content. It separates the skin from the muscles to allow for normal sliding action on each other. The superficial fascia is involved with thermoregulation, circulation, and lymphatic flow and houses the interstitium.

Looked at in diagrammatic fashion (Figure 1.4), the superficial fascia resembles nothing so much as a very strange layer cake. Of particular note are the "skin ligaments" of the retinaculum cutis superficialis. These connect to the skin and together with the superficial fascia form a three-dimensional, honeycomb-like network within the adipose layer, creating a fascial scaffold for the skin which is both flexible and resistant to mechanical load. Likewise, the retinaculum cutis profundus acts as a fascial scaffold for the deep fascia.

Deep fascia

Deep fascia is a dense, well-organized fibrous layer that covers the muscles. This is the layer that butchers and hunters refer to as the "silver skin," and for good reason (Figure 1.5). The deep fascia is sometimes referred to as the body stocking or catsuit layer (Figure 1.6), with the innermost aspect peeling away to form a discrete pocket around each muscle. This pocket is called the epimysium and serves to keep everything separate yet interconnected and, in healthy fascia, sliding on each other. The epimysium is a highly specific layer that defines both the form and volume of the underlying muscle and is the layer responsible for force transmission. So, the deep fascia includes both these individual epimysial pockets and also the broad, flat sheaths called aponeuroses that cover and connect whole groups of muscle (Figure 1.7).

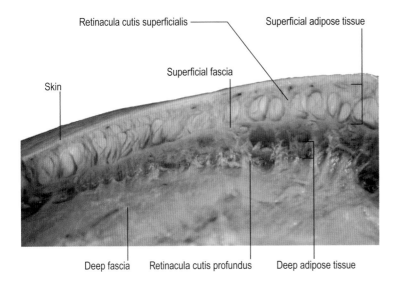

Retinacula cutis superficialis — Superficial adipose tissue

Superficial fascia

Skin

Deep fascia — Retinacula cutis profundus — Deep adipose tissue

Figure 1.3
The layers, from skin to deep fascia: The superficial fascia divides the superficial adipose tissue (SAT) from the deep adipose tissue (DAT). Note the more distinctive structure of the SAT. Its fibrous, vertically oriented membranes are somewhat regularly positioned between between lobules of fat. The DAT is much looser and irregular, with fewer fat cells. This arrangement allows for a plane of gliding between the superficial and deep fascia.
Adapted from Stecco A. et al. (2017) with permission from Handspring Publishing.

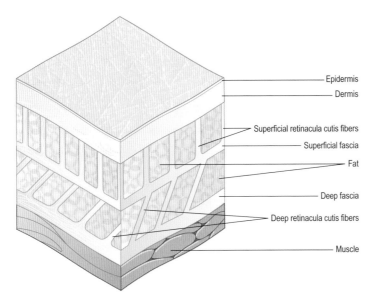

Epidermis
Dermis
Superficial retinacula cutis fibers
Superficial fascia
Fat
Deep fascia
Deep retinacula cutis fibers
Muscle

Figure 1.4
Diagram of the layers of subcutaneous tissue.
After Carla Stecco.

Use the force transmission

It is in this layer that myofascial force transmission takes place (Huijing 2009). It is well known that a muscle transmits force longitudinally across a joint, via the myotendinous junction, to create an action. So, pick up your coffee or tea and have a sip. There is a whole sequence of force transmission occurring at the shoulder, elbow, wrist joints, and fingers, and that's low impact. Imagine a right-handed baseball pitcher in the complexity of leveraging additional power from their left foot up the back of the leg to the lumbodorsal fascia to the opposite shoulder

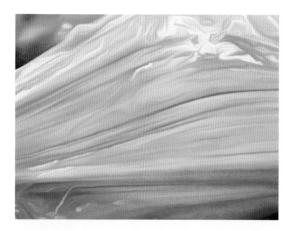

Figure 1.5
The deep fascia, or dense connective tissue, of the external oblique aponeurosis. The external oblique has been reflected from the internal oblique to expose the deep surface of its aponeurosis. Together, the aponeuroses of the external obliques, internal obliques, and transversus abdominis muscles form the strong fascial structure of the abdomen – the rectus sheath.
Photo by Nicole Trombley and Rachelle Clauson. Courtesy of AnatomySCAPES.com.

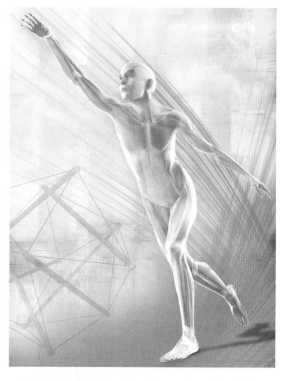

Figure 1.6
Rendering of the full body fascial "catsuit."
Illustration courtesy of fascialnet.com.

girdle (likely via the Back Functional Line, among other connections; see Chapter 3) to the right hand in order to throw a 120-mile-per-hour fast ball. And the fascia is right there along with it, transmitting that force via the epimysium (Maas & Sandercock 2010, Yucesoy 2010).

This fascial force transmission between muscles occurs in neighboring muscles, even antagonistic muscles. It is estimated that about 30 per cent of muscular tension may be transmitted in this way (Huijing et al. 2003). Would you be surprised to learn that a straight leg lift to test the hamstrings produces 2.5 times more strain in the iliotibial band than in the hamstrings (Franklyn-Miller 2009)? Understanding more about how

these interactions work should lead us to a better understanding of the pathology of chronic muscle problems, repetitive use syndromes, and more. It can also begin to explain the commonly reported phenomenon where a muscle contracting in one area can sometimes be felt very far away. As such, it is proposed that this relationship fosters reciprocal feedback between the muscles and the fascia to better regulate tension and expansion (Kwong & Findley 2014).

Meningeal fascia

Meningeal fascia surrounds the nervous system and the brain (see Chapters 4 and 5).

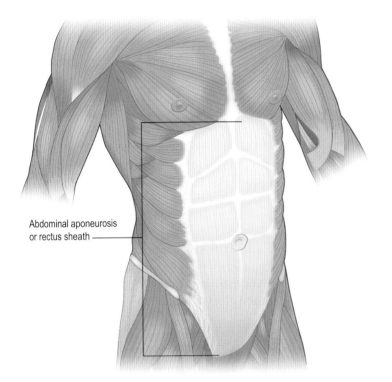

Abdominal aponeurosis
or rectus sheath

Figure 1.7
The abdominal aponeurosis – a
fascial envelope for the "six pack"
of the rectus abdominis.

Visceral fascia

Visceral fascia includes the fascia surrounding the lungs, heart, and abdominal organs. Visceral fascia suspends the organs within their cavities and includes visceral ligaments that serve to both affix the organs to the body wall and allow for physiological motion (see Chapter 6 for more details).

Viscoelasticity and the concept of "both/and"

Fascia is a colloid. Gels and emulsions are colloids. A colloid is a substance that contains particles of solid material suspended in a liquid. So, basically, a colloid is both fiber and fluid.

As a colloid, fascia exhibits a quality known as viscoelasticity. Viscoelastic materials exhibit both viscous and elastic properties when under pressure.

Elasticity is the quality of solid materials to return to their original shape after an outside force is applied to them. This is similar to pulling on a rubber band and then letting go, or, as an example of a bigger elastic deformation, similar to what one would experience after finishing a melting yoga stretch.

Viscosity is a measure of a liquid's resistance to flow. Materials with high viscosity, such as honey, move very slowly in comparison to something with low viscosity like water. High-viscosity materials seldom return to their original shape; this is called a "plastic deformation." Ever play with a piece of wet chewing gum? That is plastic deformation.

Synthetic viscoelastic materials are used in industrial applications for absorbing shock and dissipating heat. It has been shown that heating fascia decreases its viscosity, making it more fluid and moveable (Matteini et al. 2009). This strongly suggests there is good science behind warming up before working out or applying heat to a stiff area of the body.

The ability of fascia to slowly deform under load is called creep. If the load is manageable the fascia will gradually adapt to it in appropriate ways. Once that load is removed it will gradually return to its original shape, or "creep" back. This is why after sitting through a two-hour movie your buttocks do not look like the chair when you stand up. However, if the load is excessive or repeated excessively over a long period of time with no counterbalancing intervention, the fascia can become damaged.

So, fascia displays the qualities of both a solid and a liquid. But before we take a look at the "ingredients" to better understand the properties of fascia, let's travel back in time to where, or rather when, fascia begins – the womb.

In the beginning: Embryology

Fascia begins to form when the embryo is between two and three weeks old. At this point the embryo appears as a single, continuous layer of cells forming a hollow ball called the blastula. It is at about this time that the blastula begins to reorganize by folding inward on itself (invagination) and then undergoes a process called gastrulation wherein it forms into a trilaminar, three-layered disc. Some also refer to it as a trilaminar embryo (Figure 1.8):

1. Ectoderm: The upper layer, which includes the nervous system, brain, skin, and tooth enamel.

2. Mesoderm: The middle layer. This is where fascia starts. From this layer somites arise. These are groups of cells that are precursors for specialization. They will form smooth, cardiac, and skeletal muscle, mesentery, bone, cartilage, red blood cells, white blood cells, dura mater, and the notochord and microglia. Fascia develops from this layer, the mesoderm, endlessly folded and refolded initially by gastrulation and then the inherent movement of embryonic development. Or, looking at it another way, you are the most elaborate piece of origami ever.

3. Endoderm: The lower layer, from which arises the digestive system, respiratory system, liver, pancreas, and other organs, as well as the glands and organs of the endocrine system.

But is there really a trilaminar disc consisting of three distinct layers? Using "derm" (skin) implies that all three layers are epithelial in character and therefore more or less equivalent to each other, but they are not. No less an authority than *Gray's Anatomy* confirms that all three layers are not an epithelium (Standring 2005). Rather, while the endoderm and ectoderm definitively display characteristics of epithelial tissue, it may be more proper to think of the mesoderm as *mesenchyme*, embryonic connective tissue. Put another way – we have two boundary layers: the external ectoderm from which the head and limbs develop; and the internal endoderm from which the guts and organs develop. Everything else, the meso or mesenchyme, is not a discrete layer but embryonic connective tissue, or, if you like, the "tissue of innerness" (van der Wal 2021). Myself, I keep thinking about the "tissue of inbetweeness" (daswichengewebe?).

So that is where it begins, but what is fascia made of?

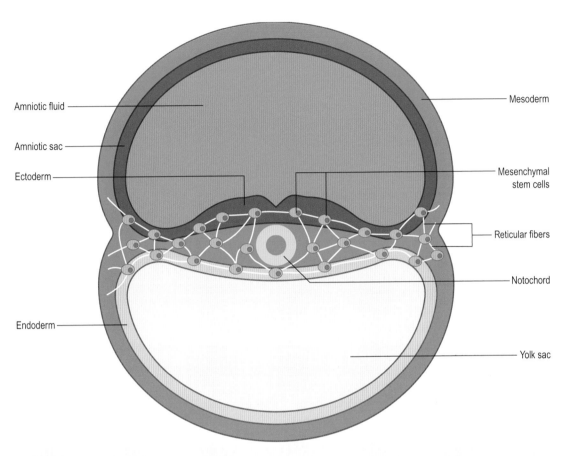

Figure 1.8
The three layers of the embryo. The middle layer, the mesoderm, forms both in between and around the endoderm and ectoderm. Fascia arises from the mesoderm, beginning as mesenchyme, loose areolar connective tissue with reticular fibers (collagen Type III).

Fascia 102

The extracellular matrix

The extracellular matrix (ECM) is "the sum total of extracellular substance within the connective tissue" (Williams 1995). That is a nice definition, but what does it really mean?

In quantum mechanics scientists posit the theory of the Higgs field, an energy field that permeates the entire universe. It is theorized that all matter in the universe arises from this field. And the confirmation, in 2012, of the existence of the Higgs boson particle brings this theory one step closer to reality.

If you look up into the night sky and contemplate the vastness and variety of the universe with all of its stars, planets, moon, nebulae, galaxies, etc., you could imagine the Higgs field as the blackness of space. Everything else – the stars, planets, moons, comets, nebulae, galaxies, and all the other matter – is supported, suspended, and generated by the invisible energy mesh of the Higgs field.

One could consider the extracellular matrix as being the Higgs field of the body. In this case, the ECM is a substrate or, more accurately, a scaffolding upon which everything else in the body is built. It is where much of the cellular matter that makes up the body is produced. It is your inner space and is no less interesting than outer space.

Of course, the other difference here is, unlike the Higgs field, we absolutely know the extracellular matrix is real. And again, the colloid ECM is a "both/and" (as opposed to either/or). The ECM is both fiber and fluid (Figure 1.9).

The fiber

The fiber of the extracellular matrix gives support and structure to the arrangement of everything in the body. It forms the scaffolding upon which the body is built and also provides mechanical linkages from cell to cell.

Collagen

The fibrous part of the fascia is largely made up of collagen, which is the most abundant protein in the body. It is non-water soluble. There are at least 15 types of collagen, but Types I, II, and III are the ones mainly found in connective tissue (Lindsay 2008).

Type I is the most abundant. It is found in the skin, bone, tendon, ligaments, and, of course, the fascia proper, and accounts for about 90 per cent of all collagen in the body (Kovanen 2002). Type II is much thinner and found in the cartilage and intervertebral discs. Both types are

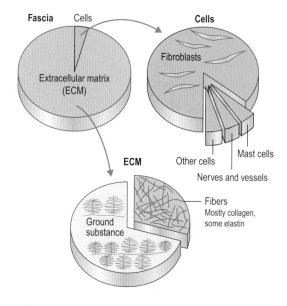

Figure 1.9

Components of fascia. The basic constituents are cells (mostly fibroblasts) and extracellular matrix (ECM), the latter of which consists of fibers plus the watery ground substance.

Illustration courtesy of fascialnet.com.

designed to resist tension but have the stretch capacity of about 10 per cent of their resting length before damage.

Type III is also found in the skin, periosteum, smooth muscle tissue, arteries, organs, and Schwann cells. The function of Type III is to provide structural maintenance to the extensile organs, wound healing, and to mediate the attachments of the tendon, ligament, and periosteum to the bone, often referred to as myotendinous junctions.

Collagen forms when molecules of tropocollagen, a more water-soluble, fragile collagen precursor, wind together to form a three-stranded helix. This triple helix of collagen fibers gives fascia tremendous tensile strength, meaning that it can be stretched without breaking (for the most part). In fact, gram for gram, Type I collagen is stronger than steel (Lodish et al. 2000), thus it can withstand tremendous force and still be able to bend with the wind. It is precisely this tensile strength that allows for plastic and elastic deformation. This is quite useful for something like a ligament.

It is also helpful for a skyscraper (Figure 1.10). The type of steel used to construct skyscrapers is known as "mild steel" in the building industry. Mild steel has the highest strength-to-weight ratio of any known building material. Also, it is highly ductile (plastic), meaning that it will not suddenly crack like porcelain or glass when subjected to extreme forces such as earthquakes. Instead, it will gradually bend out of shape and stay that way. So, we have more in common with skyscrapers than you might think.

Another vital fact about collagen is that the multiple muscle fiber bundles of the perimysium (see Chapter 3) contain about 90 per cent of all the collagen found in muscles (McCormick 1994). This location and multidirectionality of the fibers also accounts for force transmission in the fascial system (Kannus 2000, Stecco A. et al. 2015).

Collagen, bone, and fascia

Collagen is thought to follows Davis's law, a corollary to Wolff's law. Wolff's law states that bone will adapt to regular loads placed upon it, becoming stronger over time. This is a lifelong process. For example, the bones of a tennis player's racquet-holding arm are stronger than the bones of their non-racquet arm (Taylor et al. 2009) and, because they have had nothing to resist against, astronauts must undergo specific weight training to regain bone density upon returning to earth.

It is because of this property that weight training for people with osteoporosis can be so beneficial (Nelson & Wernick 2005).

Davis's law applies a similar principle to soft tissue, specifically that soft tissue will both model itself and remodel itself (in cases of injury) according to the mechanical stress it is subject to.

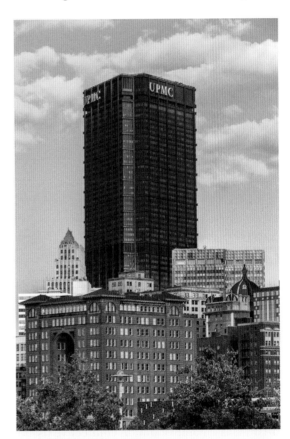

Figure 1.10
40,000 metric tons of steel comprise the 256-meter (841-ft) tall US Steel Tower in Pittsburgh, Pennsylvania. Former world headquarters of US Steel, it now houses the corporate offices of UPMC (University of Pittsburgh Medical Center).
Photo by Robert Strovers, used with kind permission.
www.robertstrovers.com

Davis's law is named after orthopedic surgeon Henry Gassett Davis (1807–1896), who was fascinated by the adaptation of soft tissue and invented a number of traction-based applications to induce soft tissue remodeling, including the first splint that would both traction and protect the hip joint.

Ligaments, or any soft tissue, when put under even a moderate degree of tension, if that tension is unremitting, will elongate by the addition of new material; on the contrary, when ligaments, or rather soft tissues, remain uninterruptedly in a loose or lax state, they will gradually shorten, as the effete material is removed, until they come to maintain the same relation to the bony structures with which they are united that they did before their shortening.

Nature never wastes her time and material in maintaining a muscle or ligament at its original length when the distance between their points of origin and insertion is for any considerable time, without interruption, shortened. (Davis 1867)

There were many such competing theories and ideas at the time, including whether or not ligaments can stretch, whether muscles contract or are merely "contractible," that muscle antagonists are a fallacy, chronic contractions were a morbidity (Kynett et al. 1862). These debates were often engaged in the service of trying to treat and understand scoliosis, and it can be no coincidence that Davis's sister suffered from severe scoliosis. In many ways these debates remind me of the hallway and after-hours discussions and arguments I often hear at symposiums. But let's move on to a different kind of charge.

Piezoelectricity is the ability of certain organic materials to generate an internal electric field in response to mechanical stress or strain. Quartz, cane sugar, and Rochelle salt all possess this quality, so do naturally occurring substances in our body, like bone. When our skeleton is under load it is the piezoelectric charge generated by that force that signals the bone-eating osteoclasts to stay away, and so the bone-building osteoblasts go to work. This results in stronger bone in the areas under load, given repetition and time, i.e., exercise. The process of a mechanical signal generating a cellular change is called mechanotransduction (see Figure 1.12). However, in the bone it is not the minerals that create the piezoelectric charge but rather the collagen that is responsible.

Similar to a common AA battery, with a positive end and a negative end, collagen fibrils exhibit a molecular dipole arrangement (Goes et al. 1999), but it is the folding, the triple-winding of helices, that makes collagen a very sensitive piezoelectric structure. It is also very sensitive to longitudinal strain. When it comes to the fibers, compression increases polarity and stretching is associated with "an overall depolarization of the system" (Ravi et al. 2012). It is precisely this tissue polarity that enables non-neuronal, sensory receptors (see Chapter 4) to detect and discern a wide variety of mechanical stimuli from their environment, for example, the pressure from the hand of a manual therapist or your body weight on a foam roller.

It should be noted that despite the research some consider this piezoelectric effect to be purely speculative (Ahn & Grodzinsky 2009). And now there are others who conclude that bone is also fascia (Levin 2021). The conclusion I draw is that while our knowledge base continues to increase and refine itself, our human nature may still be stuck in the mid-1800s. But we were discussing fiber types, weren't we? Let's get back to that.

Elastin

Thinner than collagen, elastin, as implied by its name, is an elastic fiber that adds additional resiliency to connective tissue. It is a protein that gives collagen the ability to stretch and distort. Elastin can stretch up to 230 per cent of its original length and return to its original shape. It sounds incredible but look in the mirror and tug on your ear and you will see a good example of this quality.

Another important distinction is that elastin fibers both lie at angles to and spiral around the collagen fibers, creating and reinforcing the three-dimensional flexible architecture of the fascial matrix.

Elastin can deteriorate with age and too much exposure to the sun.

Reticulin

Reticulin is formed from the much more delicate Type III collagen. Reticulin forms much of the collagen network of the organs of the body. Reticulin is also found in the fascial covering (endomysium) of each muscle fiber. We still do not know why it is there.

The fluid: The ground substance

The fluid component of ECM is called ground substance. Ground substance is a viscous, fluid environment where chemical exchanges take place in the body, and molecular exchanges between blood, lymph, and tissue cells happen. It is "the immediate environment of every cell in your body" (Juhan 2003).

Ground substance is amorphous, clear, and gelatinous. It can vary in viscoelasticity from relatively pliable loose connective tissue to more solid or turgid cartilage.

Ground substance fills the spaces between the fibers and the cells. Somewhat confusingly it is also sometimes referred to as the extrafibrillar matrix because it contains everything of the ECM except for collagen and elastin fibers. The ground substance surrounds the fascial fibers, enabling them to slide. Obviously, you need water to slide.

The ECM and water

The ECM is full of it. Water, that is. 15 liters of interstitial fluid. We are, more or less, 70 per cent water, though this percentage does change over time. While we tend to think about what we drink, we think less about what we urinate and even less about everything in between. The superficial fascia harbors 7.5 liters of that interstitial fluid. Every day those 7.5 liters of interstitial fluid wash past our cells, outside of the vascular system, mostly ending up in our lymphatics.

Interstitial fluid flow is responsible for transporting nutrients to the cells and has a role in tissue remodeling, inflammation, and lymphedema. Flow can give directional cues, driving tumor cells and lymphocytes to lymph nodes. It can also cause fibroblasts to morph into myofibroblasts (Rutkowski & Swartz 2007).

Interstitial fluid flow is vital to maintain healthy tissue; yet while very few manual therapies specifically address this, it is reasonable to conjecture that many of them do influence it regardless of their hypothesized mechanisms. There is speculation that the effectiveness of cupping and acupuncture are due to their effects on fluid flow (Yao et al. 2012), but to my mind there are potential effects from other types of manual therapy at work here, as well as another fluid aspect that needs to be addressed – the *interstitium*.

Interstitium

You might remember in the spring of 2018 almost every news source had a headline akin to "Science Discovers a New Organ." My favorite was from Buzzfeed, which read: "That 'new organ' everyone is freaking out about is probably not new." That much, at least, was accurate. To be absolutely clear, the paper that created such a fuss was entitled "Structure and distribution of an unrecognized interstitium in human tissues" (Benias et al. 2018). Note there is no mention of "new organ" in the title, nor anywhere in the paper. And yet this new discovery would prove irresistible to those versed in fascia science.

What's crucial to understanding this research and its importance is that it utilized a different way of looking at tissue biopsies – confocal laser endomicroscopy. In traditional tissue biopsies to get the tissue sample you have to cut. And every time you cut through something, no matter how precise the tool and skilled the implementer, there are always traces of that cut left in the sample. These are called artifacts. A typical biopsy image will exhibit white spaces that are thought to be tear artifacts, places where the otherwise dense collagen in the sample was microscopically torn. Rather than take an actual slice, confocal laser endomicroscopy takes an optical slice, so there is no tissue damage. These images revealed a reticular pattern in the tissue that was initially puzzling to the researchers. It did not seem to conform with the tear artifacts in a typical biopsy image. With time and study replication the researchers were able to confirm that the so-called "tear artifacts" were actually fluid-filled spaces surrounded by bundles of collagen. Everywhere they looked they found these fluid-filled spaces. "Everywhere" included the esophagus, gall bladder, small intestine, colon, urinary bladder, lungs,

stomach, periarterial and perivenular tissues and, yes, they found it in the fascia too. In fact, it bears a remarkable similarity to what we think of as the superficial fascia (Figure 1.11).

A follow-up to this study further showed this continuity (Cenaj et al. 2021). In this experiment, tattoo pigment was injected into the mesentery of the colon; and skin tissue was injected with both pigment and colloidal silver. In all cases particles of these nonbiologic substances were found quite distant from the injection sites, and across tissue boundaries traditionally thought to be impenetrable to such things. Special staining techniques showed the interstitial continuity between tissue compartments and fascial planes of the skin, colon, and liver, even down to the fibrous tissue around blood vessels (adventitia) and the perineurium of the nerves (see Chapters 6 and 4, respectively). Once again this furthered the idea of a body-wide network, a fluid-filled interstitial space. This could have profound implications on the way we treat infections and diseases like cancer. Not to mention how you feel about that tattoo you were thinking of getting.

PGs, GAGs, and HAs

Ground substance is also composed of hydrophilic proteoglycans (PGs). PGs are water-loving peptides that serve to attract water and provide a protective cushion for the ECM's collagen architecture. They are responsible for its gel-like properties. Proteoglycans are made from combinations of smaller molecules called glycosaminoglycans or GAGs.

GAGs can absorb water like a sponge. It is estimated that 90 per cent of the extracellular matrix is made up of water. GAGs, together with the strength of the collagen, help to make the ECM very good at resisting compressive forces.

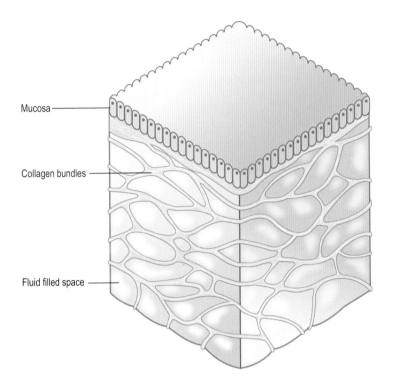

Mucosa

Collagen bundles

Fluid filled space

Figure 1.11
The schematic drawn from the Interstitium study (Benias et al. 2018), showing a fluid-filled space supported by bundles of collagen. Note the similarity of this image to Figure 1.4.

Seven distinct GAGs have so far been identified, including chondroitin and heparin. The GAG I want to focus on is hyaluronan, popularly, and inaccurately, referred to as hyaluronic acid. It is not really an acid, but the term is so pervasive now it is not likely to change, so we should be aware that these terms reference the same thing.

Hyaluronan (HA) is the most hydrophilic, water-loving of all the GAGS. It functions as the hydraulic fluid, the WD-40 that lubricates the fascia, ensuring smooth gliding between the various layers, superficial to deep, and even within the muscle tissue itself. HA is produced, predominantly, in the sliding layers between fascia and the epimysium of the muscles by a class of cells called "fasciacytes" a mechano-sensitive cell that responds to shearing motion (Stecco C. et al. 2011, 2018). The actual quantity

of hyaluronan relative to fascial tissue seems to vary with both location and function. The epimysium has six micrograms (mcg) of hyaluronan for every gram of fascial tissue, whereas the retinacula of the ankle (see Chapter 4) is one of the richest areas for HA with 90 mcg per gram of fascia (Fede et al. 2018).

Increases in the viscosity of HA are called *densifications*. This increase causes HA to become more adhesive, rather than lubricating (Pratt 2021). You get stuck instead of slide. Densifications can interfere with proper movement/body coordination. Also, given the proximal relationship of HA with certain classes of sensory nerves (see Chapter 4), densifications could shed new light on the symptomatic pain felt by so-called nerve impingements/entrapments and myofascial pain syndromes. Movement, temperature, and pH (a pH of 6.6 and under increases HA viscosity by 20 per cent) can all influence viscosity in a positive way to reduce densifications. Research into diet, pH, and a temperature, within a range of 36–40°C to minimize densification continues, as does research into the effect of manual therapy on the water content of densified hyaluronan (Menon et al. 2020).

Finally, ground substance permeates the insides of cells, as allowed by the semipermeable plasma membranes of each cell, which are governed by highly specialized cell surface receptors.

Cell receptors

Rather like individual taste buds each looking for specific flavors, cell receptors are glycoproteins arrayed along the cell membrane that are constantly monitoring the matrix. Cell receptors determine which of the many chemicals, hormones, and cytokines floating around in the ECM to take in and metabolize. The receptors do this based on their specific programming or, to keep with the metaphor, by which flavors they like. This metabolic process is essential to the health and vitality of the cell.

Many, if not most, cell receptors respond to chemical stimuli. For example, there are both CB1 and CB2 receptors in fascia (Fede et al. 2016a). A more specific study (Fede et al. 2020) stimulated endocannabinoid receptors of the principal cell-type in fascia, the fibroblast (Spoiler! See later in the chapter). It was discovered that the fibroblasts were able to rapidly (within a few hours) produce large quantities of HA and deliver it into the tissue via vesicles (fluid-filled sacs). While cannabinoids certainly can lessen the perception of pain, via the central nervous system, this shows that they have the potential to actually modify fascial tissue at the structural level.

Estrogen and relaxin also play a key role in inhibiting fibrosis and inflammatory activities within the fascia, and it has been demonstrated that fascial cells can modulate the ECM based on hormone levels (Fede et al. 2016b, 2019). Overall, low hormone levels lead to an increase in collagen Type I, which can also become more rigid during menopause. This data and other related findings shine a light on why women tend to suffer more than men, categorically, from myofascial pain.

There is another particularly fascinating receptor known as an integrin. Integrins are adhesive in nature. They stick each cell to the ECM. Furthermore, there is a continuity of fibrils from the integrin through the cell membrane all the way to the nucleus of the cell. What makes integrins unique is that they respond not to chemical stimuli but to mechanical stimuli. They are sensitive to both stretch and vibration. It is as if each cell in the body was plugged into the ECM so that it can also monitor the environment by listening to it.

When the integrin is stimulated by pressure/vibration, it responds by creating electrochemical changes that affect gene transcription. This process of creating change at the cellular level via mechanical pressure and vibration is called mechanotransduction (Figure 1.12). A study done on athletes found that vigorous massage activates mechanotransduction signaling pathways that reduced the inflammation response (Crane et al. 2012).

Mechanotransduction occurs at the speed of sound. We tend to think of the speed of sound at it relates to sound moving through the air and breaking the sound barrier. That speed is about 343 meters, or 1,125 feet, per second. That's 767 miles per hour, or 2.8 times faster than your nervous system. In water sound travels over four

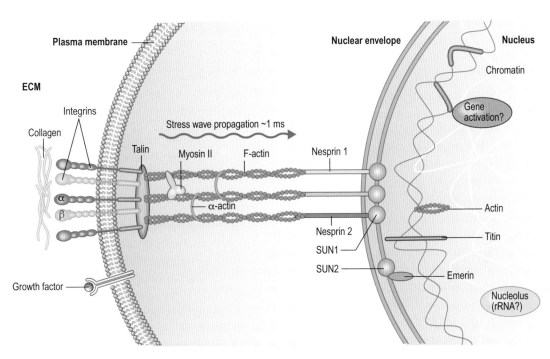

Figure 1.12

Mechanotransduction. Mechanical stimulation from the collagen fibers (Types I, III, and V) to the integrins creates a tensional pull (stress wave propagation), which cascades through the cellular cytoskeleton (talin) through the nuclear envelope to the nucleus whereupon different genes will activate and express themselves in response to the change in tension.

times faster at 1,481 meters (4,858 feet) per second. That's a little over 3,300 mph. And, as mentioned earlier, you are mostly water.

If you pull on one part of a spider's web, you can see the entire web respond. Fascia responds in much the same way. The tugs and pulls transmit information to the cells via the integrins. This in turn creates changes in chemistry, gene transcription, and even sensory perceptions (see Chapter 4).

In the simplest possible terms, the ECM is involved in every process and function of the body. It also serves as the body's intranet – a

private internal communication network. The ECM makes sure all the cells are in communication with all the other cells, creating a body-wide signaling network (Oschman 2003, Langevin 2006) that transmits mechanical signals such as strain and vibration throughout the entire organism via the fascial web.

Over enough time, persistent tension will create anomalies in the tissue. Under the best circumstances these anomalies will strengthen the tissue. Under less than optimal conditions the stress will impair the functioning of the fascia, creating compensations and, over enough time, visible distortions in posture (see Chapters 7 and 8). But what or who is the spider inside the web, responsible for maintaining the overall architecture?

The fibroblast

The fibroblast (Figure 1.13) is the most abundant cell in the fascia and it wears many hats. It is the builder, custodian, demolition squad, and EMT (Emergency Medical Technician) for the entire extracellular matrix. Fibroblasts produce all the complex carbohydrates of the ground substance. Essentially, they produce and maintain the entire extracellular matrix. Even as you sit here reading this, on a cellular level you are really quite busy. Furthermore, fibroblasts remodel their own cytoskeleton in response to changes in body position (Langevin et al. 2005). And when under a reasonable physiologic amount of stretch, fibroblasts remodel quite rapidly (seconds to minutes) and affect the stiffness and viscosity of the surrounding superficial fascia (Langevin et al. 2011). This reinforces the need for more mechanotransduction-based tissue research, and the verifiable therapeutic potentials that could arise from such studies (see Chapter 8).

Fibroblasts also synthesize and remodel all the collagen depending on the tension between the cell and the ECM. When the tension outside the cell is low, there is not much collagen production. When under high tension, the fibroblast will increase collagen production and cell proliferation (Grinnell 2007). Our movement and bodywork-based therapies, surgeries, accidents, and injuries have the potential to change the cell–ECM tension, as do our movement and manual therapies.

Fibroblasts are direction sensitive as well, and they will organize themselves based on the pull of the underlying matrix (Kirkwood & Fuller 2009). So, is it possible that the direction in which things happen, be they accidents, repetitive use, habitual movement patterns, or our therapeutic interventions, really do matter? If so, then when someone has a chronically tight and superiorly elevated shoulder girdle, as many of us do, shouldn't we orient our therapeutic interventions in a caudal or downward direction toward the sacrum?

Conversely, lack of regular movement or total immobility will give the fibroblast little to no appropriate stimulation, which will have a negative impact on the formation of a healthy collagen matrix (Figure 1.14).

So, fascia responds according to mechanical supply and demand, and follows Davis's law. Fibroblasts are both spooling out more collagen where necessary and secreting collagenase, a collagen-eating enzyme, all based on signals

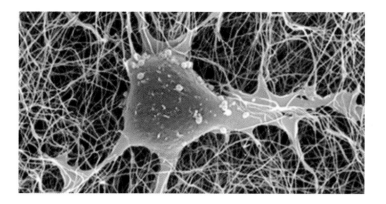

Figure 1.13

Fibroblast in the fascial net.

Reproduced from Jiang and Grinnell (2005) with permission from the American Society for Cell Biology. Available: www.molbiolcell.org/doi/10.1091/mbc.e05-01-0007 [May 18, 2022].

of pressure and vibration, like a cellular public works department – building, knocking down, and cleaning up the collagen matrix.

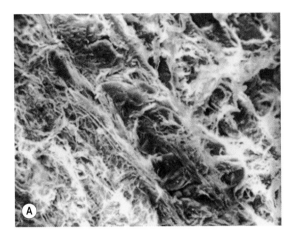

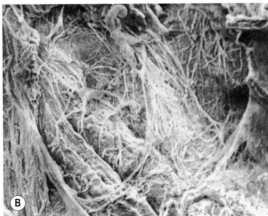

Figure 1.14

(A) This electron microscope picture shows a healthy collagen network within the fascia. (B) The same area after 3 weeks of immobilization. Note the change and disorganization in the fibers. Without proper mechanical stimulation it is as if the collagen grows like weeds, rather than a proper garden.

Reprinted by permission of Springer Nature from *Journal of Muscle Research and Cell Motility*. Organization and distribution of intramuscular connective tissue in normal and immobilized skeletal muscles. An immunohistochemical, polarization and scanning electron microscopic study. Järvinen TA, Józsa L, Kannus P, Järvinen TLN, Järvinen M 23 (3) 145–154. 2002.

Under certain conditions, fibroblasts can morph into myofibroblasts. These are the EMTs. When you are injured, they swarm to the injury site where they produce cytokines to enhance the inflammatory response (Baum & Duffy 2011). Myofibroblasts are also highly contractile, much more so than a normal fibroblast. So, when there is an open wound, they help to close that wound on a cellular level.

Even more surprising is that fibroblasts are not discrete cells. They too form an interconnected network – a web within the web (Langevin et al. 2004). Lastly, they are considered sentinel cells for the immune system. Along with producing cytokines, interleukins, and other immune function cells, it has been proposed they play a critical role in tissue inflammation and repair (Buckley 2011, Buckley et al. 2001).

Other cells

Fascia also contains T cells, mast cells, macrophages, lymphocytes, and adipocytes. Fascia also contains the recently discovered telocytes.

Telocytes

Another recently discovered cell (Popescu et al. 2011) is the telocyte. Ubiquitous in fascia throughout the body, telocytes are mechanosensitive cells that are vital to many physiological processes like stem cell upkeep, tissue repair, and immune function. Generally regarded as support cells that help maintain tissue homeostasis, telocytes are found everywhere throughout the body including in most organs and skeletal muscle tissue. They have long, finger-like, cellular extensions called telopodes. Telopodes form intricate networks within the stroma. Jargon alert: stroma. Another technical term, the stroma (also called stromal space) comprises all the parts of an organ or tissue without their specific functions. Think of a house that has all its infrastructure, plumbing, heating, but no appliances, devoid of furniture, and with no-one living in it to actuate those functions. A house but not a home. So, the stroma is the scaffolding and the ductwork. The fascia proper and ECM. Is this sounding familiar?

Anyway, back to the telocytes and their telopodes. The telocytes are communicators, and they do this by forming an intricate network of telopodes. The telocytes share intercellular information and genetic material via extracellular vesicles (EVs), which are amorphous, cellular blobs that emerge from the telopodes and shuttle information to nearby cells. As such, telocytes are major players in intercellular communication. Along with the fibroblast network, telocytes lend additional credence to the idea that fascia forms a body-wide, cellular signaling network (Langevin 2006, Oschman 2003). EVs are also thought to have an important role in maladies like cancer and neurodegenerative and cardiovascular diseases.

At the vanguard of regenerative medicine research, telocytes are thought to be part of stem cell niches – the microenvironment around the stem cell (Rosa et al. 2021).

Fascia 103

To reiterate, from the fascial point of view, everything is both separate and interconnected. But the reality under the skin is not so simple. In fact, it is very far from simple.

Under the endoscope

On the outskirts of the city of Bordeaux in France lies the L'Institut Aquitain de la Main (The Aquitaine Institute of the Hand). It is a plain and unassuming building, so much so that the first time I was there I drove right past it – and kept on driving right past it again and again (this was

pre-GPS) – until it made me quite late for my formal meeting with Dr. Jean-Claude Guimberteau.

I had first met Dr. Guimberteau in 2007 at the First Fascia Research Congress. He was there debuting his groundbreaking fascial research. When I saw him all by himself in an elevator I decided that wherever he was going I was going there too.

A tendon transplant surgeon, Dr. Guimberteau embarked on a quest to better understand how the tendons slide on each other. Using an endoscopic camera with a general magnification of $25 \times$, but capable of $65 \times$, he produced the first in vivo pictures and videos of the living fascial system (Figure 1.15). He did not understand what he was seeing. The anatomy books and the cadaver lab make it very simple and linear. What Dr. Guimberteau found was not linear. It seemed disorganized and chaotic. At first it seemed illogical to his Cartesian way of thinking that such chaos and efficiency could coexist so perfectly, but rather than being daunted by it Dr. Guimberteau was to devote his life to exploring and trying to understand it.

Most of all he was struck by the continuity of it all:

There is no break in the tissue continuity, be it within muscle, tendons, or around the arterial and venous structures and the structures surrounding the adipocytes. All these structures are formed in the same manner and are continuous. We have discovered the same continuity of tissue within the sub-cutaneous tissue…the epidermis and dermis and the muscles.

The concept of the organization of living matter into stratified layers, hierarchical layers of sheaths, lamellae and strata cannot satisfy an anatomist who studies precise, endoscopic, functional anatomy. Even though they may be of different colours, textures and shapes, they are all linked to each other. This is a global tissue concept. (Guimberteau 2016)

Here was a brave, new fibrillar world. A beautiful, fractal realm where opalescent fibers continuously change and reform, based on the tension of the moment (Figure 1.16). Yet for all this apparent lack of coherent order in the fascia, there was no doubt it allowed for the efficient moving and gliding of the adjacent structures (Figure 1.17). Dr. Guimberteau named this sliding system the Multimicrovacuolar Collagenic Absorbing System. The microvacuoles are formed by microfibrils 10 to 100 micrometers in length (note: 1 micrometer = 1 millionth of a meter). These infinitesimal fibers, predominantly collagen Types I and III, create polyhedral shapes,

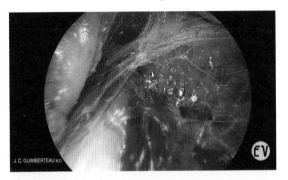

Figure 1.15
There are no empty spaces in the body. All available space is occupied (5 ×).
Reproduced with the kind permission of Endovivo Productions and J.-C. Guimberteau M.D.

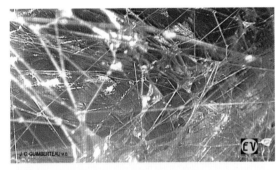

Figure 1.16
A world of fibers exists in every nook and cranny (65 ×).
Reproduced with the kind permission of Endovivo Productions and J.-C. Guimberteau M.D.

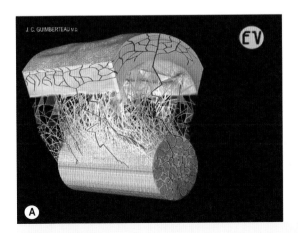

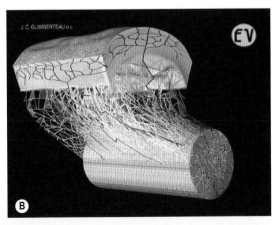

Figure 1.17
Computer diagrams of the sliding system illustrating no breakage in continuity.
Reproduced with the kind permission of Endovivo Productions and J.-C. Guimberteau M.D.

which enclose the microvacuole (Figure 1.18). The microvacuole is filled with a glycosaminoglycan (GAG) gel.

Like snowflakes, no two microvacuoles are the same. Geometrically, they are fractals (Figure 1.19). Fractals are seemingly never-ending

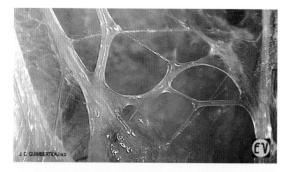

Figure 1.18
The microvacuole: the intersection of fibrils in three dimensions that form an irregular polyhedral unit of volume (130 ×).
Reproduced with the kind permission of Endovivo Productions and J.-C. Guimberteau M.D.

patterns, wherein even the smallest parts reflect the general shape of the whole. This property is called self-similarity. Seashells and snowflakes are fractal. Not limited to geometry, fractal patterns have been found in sound, and some theorists propose that fractals can even describe processes in time.

Fractal mathematics is quite useful in modeling the structure of things that seem random in pattern, but have an inherent, implicate order, for example, eroding coastlines, crystal growth, fluid turbulence, and even the formation of galaxies.

We have spent so much time studying the cells that we have completely ignored the environment that surrounds the cells. We have discovered and named all the trees insofar as we know, but at last we can see the whole forest. And there is a whole other universe in that forest.

Perhaps it is time to start rethinking the way we think the human body is structured.

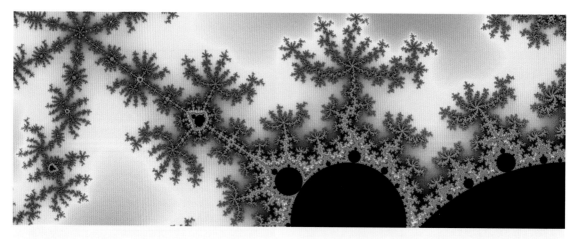

Figure 1.19
A typical fractal, where every smaller section of the image reflects the overall pattern of the whole image.
Courtesy of Creative Commons (https://creativecommons.org/licenses/by-sa/4.0).

References

Adstrum S (2014) Fascial eponyms may help elucidate terminological and nomenclatural development. J Bodywork Mov Ther. July; 19 (3) 516–525.

Ahn A C and Grodzinsky A J (2009) Relevance of collagen piezoelectricity to "Wolff"'s Law": A critical review. Med Eng Phys. September; 31 (7) 733–741.

Baum J and Duffy H S (2011) Fibroblast and myofibroblasts: What are we talking about? J Cardiovasc Pharmacol. April; 57 (4) 376–379.

Benias P C, Wells, R G, Sackey-Aboagye B et al. (2018) Structure and distribution of an unrecognized interstitium in human tissues. March; Sci Rep 8, 4947.

Buckley C D (2011) Why does chronic inflammation persist: An unexpected role for fibroblasts. Immunol Lett. July; 138 (1) 12–14.

Buckley C D, Piling D, Lord J M et al. (2001) Fibroblasts regulate the switch from acute resolving to chronic persistent inflammation. Trends Immunol. April; 22 (4) 199–204.

Cenaj O, Allison D H R, Imam R et al. (2021) Evidence for continuity of interstitial spaces across tissue and organ boundaries in humans. Commun Biol. March; 4 (1) 436.

Crane J D, Ogborn D I, Cupido C et al. (2012) Massage therapy attenuates inflammatory signaling after exercise-induced muscle damage. Sci Transl Med. February; 4 (119) 119ra13.

Davis H G (1867) Conservative Surgery as Exhibited in Remedying some of the Mechanical Causes that Operate Injuriously both in Health and Disease. New York, NY: D. Appleton & Company.

Fede C, Albertin G, Petrelli L et al. (2016a) Expression of endocannabinoid receptors in human fascial tissue. Eur J Histochem. June; 60 (2) 2643.

Fede C, Albertin G, Petrelli L et al. (2016b) Hormone receptor expression in human fascial tissue. Eur J Histochem. November; 60 (4) 2710.

Fede C, Angelini A, Stern R et al. (2018) Quantification of hyaluronan in human fasciae: Variations with function and anatomical site. J Anat. October; 233 (4) 552–556.

Fede C, Pirri C, Fan C et al. (2019) Sensitivity of the fasciae to sex hormone levels: Modulation of collagen-I, collagen-III and fibrillin production. PLOS ONE. September; 14 (9) e0223195.

Fede C, Pirri C, Petrelli L et al. (2020) Sensitivity of the fasciae to the endocannabinoid system: Production of hyaluronan-rich vesicles and potential peripheral effects of cannabinoids in fascial tissue. Int J Mol Sci. April; 21 (8) 2936.

Findley T W and Schleip R (eds) (2007) Introduction. Fascia Research: Basic Science and Implications for Conventional and Complementary Health Care. Munich: Elsevier Urban and Fischer, p. 2.

Franklyn-Miller A, Falvey E C, Clark R et al. (2009) The strain patterns of the deep lower limb. Fascia Research II: Basic Science and Implications for Conventional and Complimentary Care. Munich: Elsevier GmbH.

Fricker M D, Heaton L M, Jones, N S and Boddy L (2021) The mycelium as a network. Microbiol Spectr. May; 5 (3); doi: 10.1128/microbiolspec. FUNK-0033-2017.

Garfin S R, Tipton C M, Mubarak S J et al. (1981) Role of fascia in maintenance of muscle tension and pressure. J Appl Physiol Respir Environ Exerc Physiol. August; 51 (2) 317–320.

Goes J C, Figueiro S D, De Pavia J A C and Sombra A S B (1999) Piezoelectric and dielectric properties of collagen films. Phys Status Solidi. October; 176 (2) 1077–1083.

Grinnell F (2007) Fibroblast mechanics in three-dimensional collagen matrices [DVD recording]. First International Fascia Research Congress, Boston, Mass.

Guimberteau J-C (2016) An interview with Dr. Jean-Claude Guimberteau, January 7, 2016. [Online] Available: www.fascialfitness.net.au/articles/an-interview-with-dr-jean-claude-guimberteau [May 23, 2022].

Huijing P A (2009) Epimuscular myofascial force transmission: A historical review and implications for new research. International Society of Biomechanics Muybridge Award Lecture, Taipei, 2007. J Biomech. January; 42 (1) 9.

Huijing P A, Maas H and Baan G C (2003) Compartmental fasciotomy and isolating a muscle from neighboring muscles interfere with myofascial force transmission within the rat anterior crural compartment. J Morphol. March; 256 (3) 306–321.

Järvinen T A, Józsa L, Kannus P et al. (2002) Organization and distribution of intramuscular connective tissue in normal and immobilized skeletal muscles. An immunohistochemical, polarization and scanning electron microscopic study. J Muscle Res Cell Motil. 23 (3) 245–254.

Jiang H and Grinnell F (2005) Cell–matrix entanglement and mechanical anchorage of fibroblasts in three-dimensional collagen matrices. Mol Biol Cell. November; 16 (11) 5070–5076.

Juhan D (2003) Job's Body, 3rd edn. Barrytown, NY: Barrytown/Station Hill Press Inc.

Kannus P (2000) Structure of the tendon connective tissue. Scan J Med Sci Sports. 10 (6) 312–320.

Kirkwood J E and Fuller G G (2009) Liquid crystal collagen: A self-assembled morphology for the orientation of mammalian cells. Langmuir (ACS Publications). February; 25 (5) 3200–3206.

Kovanen V (2002) Intramuscular extracellular matrix: Complex environments of muscle cells. Exerc Sport Sci Rev. January; 30 (1) 20–25.

Kumka M and Bonar J (2012) Fascia: A morphological description and classification system based on literature review. J Can Chiropr Assoc. September; 56 (3) 179–191.

Kwong E H and Findley T W (2014) Fascia—current knowledge and future directions in physiatry: Narrative review. J Rehabil Res Dev. 51 (6) 875–884.

Kynett H H, Butler S W and Brinton D G (1862). Medical and Surgical Reporter. 8. p. 518.

Langevin H M (2006) Connective tissue: A body-wide signaling network? Med Hypotheses. February; 66 (6) 1074–1077.

Langevin H M, Bouffard N, Badger G J et al. (2005) Dynamic fibroblast cytoskeletal response to subcutaneous tissue stretch ex vivo and in vivo. Am J Physiol Cell Physiol 288 C747–C756.

Langevin H M, Bouffard N, Fox J R et al. (2011) Fibroblast cytoskeletal remodeling contributes to connective tissue tension. J Cell Physiol. May; 226 (5) 1166–1175.

Langevin H M, Cornbrooks C J and Taatjes D J (2004) Fibroblasts form a body-wide cellular network. Histochem Cell Biol. July; 122 (1) 7–15.

Levin S M (2021) Bone is fascia. In: Lowell de Solórzano S. Everything Moves: How Biotensegrity Informs Human Movement. Edinburgh: Handspring Publishing, pp 35–39.

Lindsay M (2008) Fascia: Clinical Applications for Health and Human Performance. Clifton Park, NY: Delmar.

Lodish H, Berk A, Zipursky S L et al. (2000) Molecular Cell Biology, 4th edn. New York, NY: W H Freeman.

Maas H and Sandercock T G (2010) Force transmission between synergistic skeletal muscles through connective tissue linkages. J Biomed Biotechnol. February; Volume 2010 ID 575672.

Matteini P, Dei L, Carretti E et al. (2009) Structural behavior of highly concentrated hyaluronan. Biomacromolecules. June; 10 (6) 1516–1522.

McCormick R J (1994) The flexibility of the collagen compartment of muscle. Meat Sci. 36(1/2) 79–91.

Menon R, Oswald S, Raghavan P et al. (2020) T1ρ-mapping for musculoskeletal pain diagnosis: Case series of variation of water bound glycosaminoglycans quantification before and after Fascial Manipulation® in subjects with elbow pain. Int J Environ Res Public Health. January; 17 (3) 708.

Nelson M and Wernick S (2005) Strong Women Stay Young. New York: Bantam Books.

Oschman J (2003) Connective tissue as an energetic and informational continuum. Structural Integration. August; 31 (3) 5–15.

Pratt R (2021) Hyaluronan and the fascial frontier. Int J Mol Sci. June; 22 (13) 6845.

Popescu L M, Manole E, Şerboiu C et al. (2011) Identification of telocytes in skeletal muscle interstitium: Implication for muscle regeneration. J Cell Mol Med. June; 15 (6) 1379–1392.

Ravi H K, Simona F, Hulliger J and Cascella M (2012) Molecular origin of piezo- and pyroelectric properties in collagen investigated by molecular dynamics simulations. J Phys Chem B. February; 116 (6) 1901–1907.

Rosa I, Marini M and Manetti M (2021) Telocytes: An emerging component of stem cell niche microenvironment. J Histochem Cytochem. December; 69 (12) 795–818.

Rutkowski J M and Swartz M A (2007) A driving force for change: Interstitial fluid flow as a morphoregulator. Trends Cell Biol. January; 17 (1) 44–50.

Schleip R (2005) Active fascial contractility: Fascia may be able to contract in a smooth muscle-like manner and thereby influence musculoskeletal dynamics. Med Hypothesis. 65 (2) 273–277.

Schleip R, Hedley G and Yucesoy C A (2019) Fascial nomenclature: Update on related consensus process. Clin Anat. October; 32 (7) 929–933.

Schleip R, Klingler W and Lehmann-Horn F (2006) Fascia is able to contract in a smooth muscle-like manner and thereby influence musculoskeletal mechanics. J Biomech. 39 (Supplement 1) S488.

Standring S (ed.) (2005) Gray's Anatomy: The Anatomical Basis of Clinical Practice, 39th edn. Edinburgh: Elsevier Churchill Livingstone.

Stecco A, Busoni F, Stecco C et al. (2015) Comparative ultrasonographic evaluation of the Achilles paratenon in symptomatic and asymptomatic subjects: An imaging study. Surg Radiol Anat. April; 37 (3) 281–285.

Stecco A, Stecco C and Stecco L (2017) The superficial fascia. In: Liem T, Tozzi P, and Chila A (eds.) (2017) Fascia in the Osteopathic Field. Edinburgh, UK: Handspring Publishing.

Stecco C (2015) Anatomy consensus in nomenclature. 2015 Fascia Research Congress Video. [Online] Available: www.fasciaresearchsociety.org/congress_recordings_proceeding.php [May 23, 2022].

Stecco C, Fede C, Macchi V et al. (2018) Fasciacytes: A new cell devoted to fascial gliding regulation. Clin Anat. March; 31 (5) 667–676.

Stecco C, Stern R, Porzionato A et al. (2011) Hyaluronan within fascia in the etiology of myofascial pain. Surg Radiol Anat. December; 33 (10) 891–896.

Taylor R E, Zheng C, Jackson R P et al. (2009) The phenomenon of twisted growth: Humeral torsion in dominant arms of high performance tennis players. Comput Methods Biomech Biomed Engin. February; 12 (1) 83–89.

van der Wal J (2021) De Fabrica Humani Corporis – Fascia as the Fabric of the Body. In: Lesondak D and Akey A M (eds) Fascia, Function, and Medical Applications. pp 13–14. Boca Raton, FL: CRC Press/ Taylor & Francis.

Varela F J and Frenk S (1987) The organ of form: Towards a theory of biological shape. Journal of Social Biology and Structure. 10 (1) 73–83.

Vleeming A (2011) Comment made by Vleeming in symposia where this author was also presenting. September, 2011, Manchester, UK.

Williams P (ed.) (1995) Gray's Anatomy: The Anatomical Basis of Medicine and Surgery, 38th edn. Edinburgh, UK: Churchill Livingstone, p. 75.

Yao W, Li Y, Ding G (2012) Interstitial fluid flow: The mechanical environment of cells and foundation of meridians. Evid Based Complement and Alternat Med. 2012 853516.

Yucesoy C A (2010) Epimuscular myofascial force transmission implies novel principles for muscular mechanics. Exerc Sport Sci Rev. July; 38 (3) 128–134.

Further reading

Bei Y, Wang F, Yang C and Xiao J (2015) Telocytes in regenerative medicine. J Cell Mol Med. July; 19 (7) 1441–1454.

Blechschmidt E (2004) The Ontogenetic Basis of Human Anatomy: A Biodynamic Approach to Development from Conception to Birth. Berkeley, CA: North Atlantic Books.

Chaitow L (ed.) (2014) Fascial Dysfunction. Edinburgh, UK: Handspring Publishing.

Chila A (Executive Editor) (2011) Foundations of Osteopathic Medicine. Baltimore & Philadelphia: Lippincott Williams & Wilkins.

Guimberteau J-C and Armstrong C (2015) Architecture of Human Living Fascia: The Extracellular Matrix and Cells Revealed Through Endoscopy. Edinburgh, UK: Handspring Publishing.

Krauss L (2012) A Universe from Nothing: Why There is Something Rather Than Nothing. New York, NY: Atria/Simon & Schuster.

Lesondak D and Akey A (eds) (2021) Fascia, Function, and Medical Applications. Boca Raton, FL: CRC Press/Taylor & Francis.

Myers T W (2014) Anatomy Trains: Myofascial Meridians for Manual & Movement Therapists, 3rd edn. Edinburgh, UK: Elsevier.

Pischinger A (2007) The Extracellular Matrix and Ground Regulation: Basis for a Holistic Biological Medicine. Berkeley, California: North Atlantic Books.

Schleip R, Findley T W, Chaitow L and Huijing P A (eds) (2012) Fascia: The Tensional Network of the Human Body. Edinburgh, UK: Churchill Livingstone Elsevier.

Stecco C (2015) Functional Atlas of the Human Fascial System. Edinburgh, UK: Churchill Livingstone Elsevier.

2

Fascia, Tensegrity, and the Cell

There is no real difference between structure and function; they are two sides of the same coin. If structure does not tell us something about function, it means we have not looked at it correctly.

—Andrew Taylor Still, 1899

Introduction

Why does every documentary about the human body begin with something like: "The human body is the most complex *machine* ever created"? The human body is not a machine. While it is complex – there is no denying that – the body is a complex, biodynamic, self-regulating *organism*. As much as the body is substance and matter, it is also made up of systems and processes that grow and unfold from a single cell to an embryo, and then to an adult.

Visit Ulm, Germany, and one can see some surprisingly elegant examples of artificial limbs dating back to the 1700s (Figure 2.1). It seems we humans have always had the need – perhaps it is an instinct – to replace that which we have lost. And as technology increases, so too does the sophistication of our replacement parts – and this is good. But is there a danger to thinking about the body as being a collection of parts that can be replaced or upgraded at any time?

Anyone who has ever delayed repairing their car, whether out of ignorance or financial inability to do so, knows what I am talking about here. Delay the solution long enough and soon replacing a simple part becomes a complex and more expensive repair job as other parts or systems of

the car are affected by irregular wear. Or perhaps the patient rejects the transplant. I once replaced a bad transmission – a vital organ of my automobile. It was through my own neglect that my car needed the surgery in the first place. My surgeon – I mean mechanic – cautioned me that it was a rebuilt transmission and might not last more than six months. And that is about how long it lasted. I wound up replacing the entire car. That was an easy, if expensive, solution. We cannot. however, replace our entire body.

Like many of you, I have treated patients who have undergone, or are about to undergo, a very necessary surgery, or worked with them to delay or ameliorate a probable surgery in the future. And while this is worthy work to be doing, it is nonetheless great that we live in a time where we can replace knees and hips, transplant livers and hearts, and do these things with relative efficiency and reasonably predictable outcomes.

I have also treated patients who are resigned to the fact that they will have to get replacement knees, or hips, or whatever, eventually because "that is what happens when you get old." Strangely, that did not happen to my grandmother, who lived to be 88 years old and died of "natural causes." Certainly, in her eighties things for my grandma were not what they used to be in her

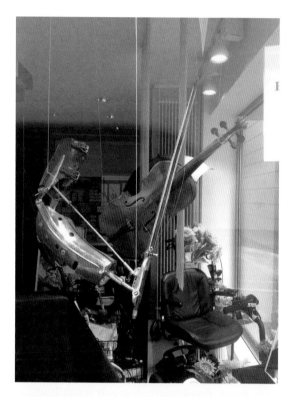

Figure 2.1
Examples of artificial limbs dating back to the 1700s.
Photo by author.

vigorous, hard-working youth, but neither did she suffer from any serious deteriorating musculoskeletal conditions.

I have also treated patients for whom the replacement joint failed, or did not quite work correctly, or whose augmentation surgeries had unintentionally painful side effects, and many more patients whose multiple orthopedic surgeries failed to relieve their symptomatic pain. So, what went "wrong" for these people? Why didn't the replacement parts work? What should we make of those cases?

And what should we make of a recent study (Försh et al. 2016) showing no clinical benefits

for patients who had spinal decompression surgery (where a small piece of bone over the nerve root, and/or some disc material is removed to create more space for healing, common forms being microdiscectomy and laminectomy) compared with patients who had spinal decompression surgery with the addition of a spinal fusion?

While it is mechanically important to get that replacement knee to bend to 110 degrees of flexion within a reasonable time after surgery, how we get there is equally important to the process of how the body needs to function as a whole. Just because the knee can be forced to bend to 110 degrees this is not an indicator of the pliability of the tissue, or resiliency with respect to the whole leg. My own experience often points to faster results by working with patients considerably upstream or downstream from the replacement joint.

Where we often fail is in not fully integrating parts with process and expecting the body to behave in a precisely linear fashion. When it does not, and this is often the case, how many clinicians and physicians are quick to blame the patient, rather than look for a reasonable alternative?

And how did we arrive at this place?

The origins of biomechanics

In 1680, Giovanni Alfonso Borelli, the father of biomechanics, published *De Motu Animalium I*. In this volume (and its sequel, *De Motu Animalium II*), Borelli equated the bodies of animals and humans to machines that function as an intricate system of beams, pulleys, and levers, using mathematics to prove his theories about how the body functions (Figure 2.2). Pick up any physical therapy textbook and one

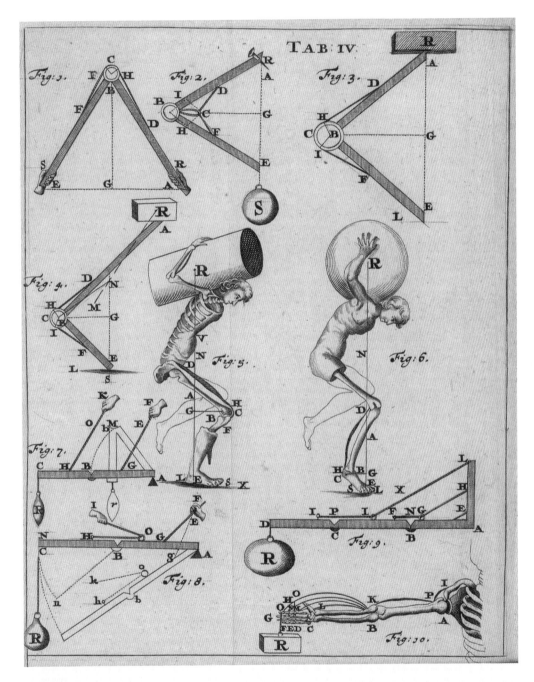

Figure 2.2
Borelli's Lever Man. Illustration from *De Motu Animalium*, 1685, by Giovanni Alfonso Borrelli (1608–1679). *IC6 B6447 680db, Houghton Library, Harvard University. Public domain {{PD-US}}.

can see a picture that models the human elbow as a simple lever and pulley (Figure 2.3). I am not disputing that ostensibly simple, functional design but the elbow does not function in isolation. What happens when that elbow joint is under load, for example, during weightlifting or when picking up a small child?

First the fingers flex to grip the load. The eight bones of the wrist stabilize, and the ligaments of the elbow joint engage, as do the various muscles and fascia that comprise the arm, shoulders, and neck. Then add having to bend the low back and perhaps bend the knees or flex the hips, depending on the size of the load. When we get to this level of complexity of movement the relationship between stability and movement begin to change more quickly than partners in a line dance.

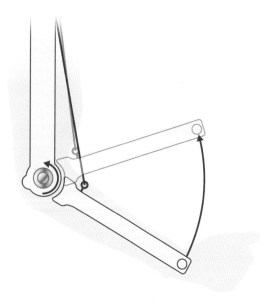

Figure 2.3
The human elbow as a simple lever and pulley.

Let's simplify this a little by considering the wrist joint under load. The conventional understanding is that the eight bones of the wrist joint temporarily fuse until the wrist is no longer under load. Pick up a heavy weight and they definitely feel like they do, so that has to be right, doesn't it?

Actually, it is wrong. In its simplest terms, the calculated forces required to achieve such a feat would tear ligaments and muscles, crush wrist bones, and exhaust your energy (Gracovetsky 2008, Levin 2011). You would have a total system failure. Similar explanations are still used for lifting heavy objects. Many of us still labor under incorrect assumptions about how the back muscles are involved in lifting, for example, in the erector spinae group. It has been calculated that the maximum force the erector spinae can endure is about 50 kilograms. Since it is possible to lift much heavier objects than that it was proposed that intra-abdominal pressure lifts the diaphragm and supports the additional weight (Bartelink 1957). There is math, however, that shows one unfortunate side effect for power lifters. At weights in excess of 200 kilos, not uncommon, that much intra-abdominal pressure would cause you to explode (Gracovetsky 2008).

The incorrect assumption here is that living organisms function in the same way as machines or inanimate materials. That is because the rules of classical physics were discovered through experiments involving inanimate objects and we have transferred those principles to living biological systems, expecting them to behave the same way. Does it make sense, evolutionarily speaking, for biological life to have modeled itself on machines that hadn't been invented yet?

The stress–strain curve is a mathematical formula that shows how much the amount of force (stress) causes an object under that stress to lengthen (strain). Stress and strain have a linear relationship. This is the case with inanimate matter, think of manmade things such as steel. Not so with viscoelastic materials, think of pulling taffy. Biological organisms can become stronger when under stress, or load, with certain aspects of the organism stiffening while under that load. Some aspects can expand and grow larger when stretched, like your Achilles tendon – a quality known as auxetic (Gatt et al. 2015). Bones and tendons can store large amounts of energy when under this load and return it with even more force, like an elastic spring (Biewener 1998, Kawakami et al. 2002).

Likewise, Galileo's Square-Cube Law helps us to build skyscrapers that do not fall down, and to understand why they are harder to build as the building gets taller. The Square-Cube Law states that as a shape grows in size, its volume increases faster than its surface area, but when that same principle is applied to a Brontosaurus, the poor dinosaur would collapse under its own weight (Scarr 2014). Increasingly, it is believed that the Square-Cube Law works fine for building inanimate objects, like buildings, but is not adequate to explain biological organisms.

Clearly, something else must be at work here.

Tensegrity – the something else

One day Dr. Stephen Levin was at the Smithsonian National Museum of Natural History in Washington, DC. He was staring at the fossilized skeleton of a Brontosaurus (Figure 2.4). Or was it an Apatosaurus? Science is still trying to figure that one out, too (Choi 2015).

Anyway, Levin was regarding this sauropod's 15-meter (50-feet) long neck, considering its cervical thoracic junction, and the size of its leg bones, and reached the conclusion that no way could the biomechanics of such a massive, complex, and frankly, ridiculous creature be explained by the classical physics beam, pulley, and lever model. You could almost say he felt the truth of it in his bones.

A successful orthopedic surgeon, Dr. Levin was deeply disturbed by this sudden revelation. It filled him with doubt about everything

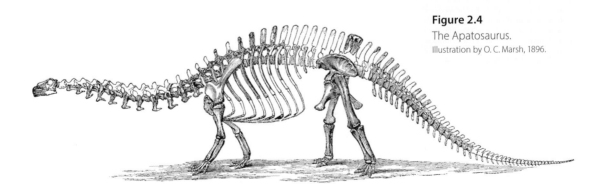

Figure 2.4
The Apatosaurus.
Illustration by O. C. Marsh, 1896.

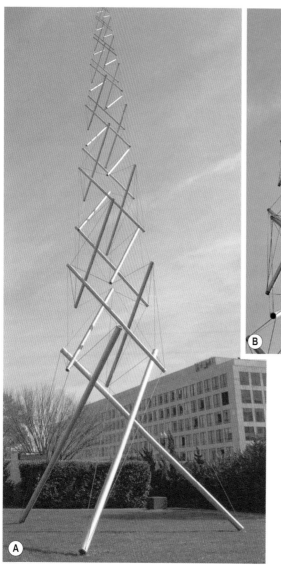

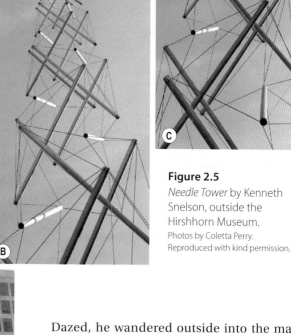

Figure 2.5
Needle Tower by Kenneth Snelson, outside the Hirshhorn Museum.
Photos by Coletta Perry.
Reproduced with kind permission.

he had been taught about how the human body was put together and how it functioned. If all of that was wrong, or at least horribly over-simplified, was there even a reason for him to perform surgeries anymore?

Dazed, he wandered outside into the mall. Suddenly he came across a sculpture that stopped him dead in his tracks. Known as *Needle Tower* (Figure 2.5), it was a very tall sculpture, with a height of 18.2 meters (60 feet), certainly on par with the size of the dinosaur that troubled him so. The sculpture was made of aluminum rods that gleamed in the afternoon sun, but what attracted Dr. Levin's attention was how none of these massive members actually touched each other. The compressive force of the rods was held in place by tension generated by a contiguous network of heavy wires. The wires elegantly suspend the rods and together distribute the force throughout the whole system. In engineering this is known as *prestress*, a way of creating both buildings and building materials that are better suited to withstand tensile forces. In the art world this structure is known as a floating compression sculpture (Figure 2.6) and it would forever change Dr. Levin's concept of the human form.

Floating compression sculptures were invented by the artist Kenneth Snelson (Figure 2.7). He built the first simple prototype when he was but a student, giving it to his favorite professor – designer, inventor, author, and systems theorist Buckminster Fuller.

Intriguingly, that prototype and the term "floating compression sculpture," by and large disappeared. What arose in its place was the term "tensegrity," and from that developed the most familiar of any of Fuller's inventions – the geodesic dome (Figure 2.8).

Sturdy as they are flexible, tensegrity structures have incredible tensile strength, withstand tremendous forces, and hold their inherent shape. "Tensegrity" is a portmanteau, a combination

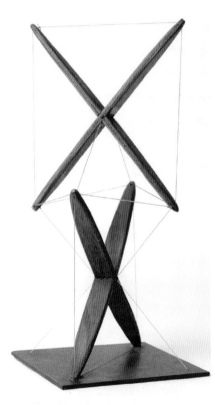

Figure 2.6
Early X-Piece, 1948, wood and nylon. Sculpture by Kenneth Snelson.
Reproduced with permission.

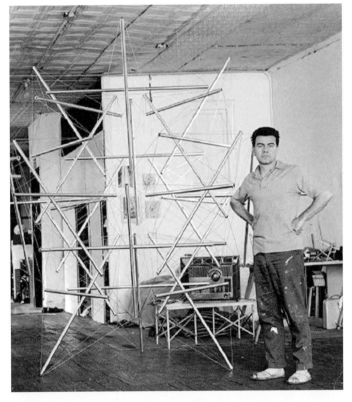

Figure 2.7
Kenneth Snelson, the artist in his studio with tensegrity sculpture, 1960.
Reproduced with permission.

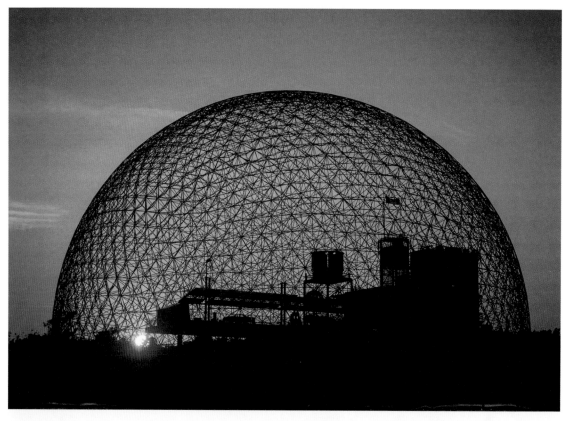

Figure 2.8
Geodesic dome designed by Buckminster Fuller for the Montreal Expo in 1967 at Parc Jean-Drapeau.
Courtesy of Guilherme Garcia and Creative Commons (https://creativecommons.org/licenses/by-sa/3.0/deed.en).

of the words, "tension" and "integrity." Fuller's definition reads as follows: "Any structure that employs contiguous tension members and discontinuous compression members in such a way that each member operates with maximum efficiency and economy."

The definition of tensegrity may be a mouthful to a non-engineer, Snelson himself did not care for the term. He likened it to "the name of a bad breakfast cereal" (Snelson 2013). An easy way to think about tensegrity is when push and

pull have a win–win relationship with each other (Figure 2.9).

Another example of a tensegrity structure (one of Fuller's favorites) is a simple balloon. In a balloon, the outer surface continuously pulls while inside the balloon the air molecules discontinuously push against it from inside. All external forces are distributed throughout the entire balloon, and we all know how hard it is to break a balloon (outside of pins or sudden, blunt trauma).

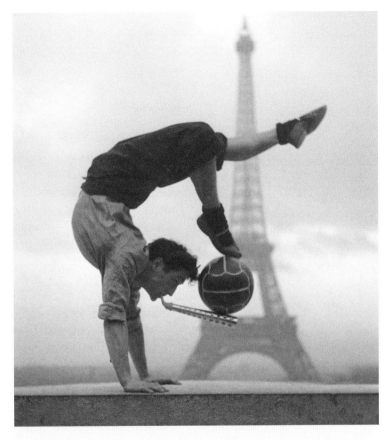

Figure 2.9
Acrobat in front of the Eiffel Tower, January 1948.
Getty Images.

Going back to pick on classical physics (do not take it personally, classical physicists!), the models we have for the human body are based on a square-frame design.

Right now, look at your house or the room that you are in. These are examples of square-frame design. It is not an inherently bad design, but it does take a lot of support, beaming, and bracing to hold it up and resist gravity. And while very solid, square-frame designs are not terribly resilient (Figure 2.10).

Square-frame design has no spring to it at all. No bounce. Thank God we humans do.

Compared with its square brethren, the essential "building block" of a tensegrity structure is not a block at all. It is a triangle, specifically a three-dimensional triangle known as a truss (think of a pyramid instead of a cube). The unique thing about a truss design is, unlike a square-frame house, it evenly distributes strain throughout the entire structure. When a tensegrity structure is compressed, there is no linear stress–strain curve.

The structure absorbs the stress and then returns to its shape when the stress is removed. In essence, it bounces back.

The architect, Eero Saarinen, who designed the Gateway Arch in St. Louis (Figure 2.11), and the engineers who built it surely understood this. The Gateway Arch is the tallest arch in the world, topping out at 192 meters (630 feet) at its apex. Although not technically a tensegrity structure, and not apparent from the outside either, it is a giant, hollow truss. More specifically, it is a giant, stainless steel hollow truss, with each triangular piece varying slightly from one to the next, interlocking to hold the Arch upright. Interestingly, these trusses are held together not just by welds and compression, but also by the tension of long steel cables, referred to by the builders of the arch as "tendons." All part of the Arch's prestress.

This engineering marvel makes the arch earthquake resistant. It can also withstand winds of up to 150 miles per hour, with the ability to sway 46 centimeters (18 inches) in either direction.

That is amazingly resilient, and more like our own amazingly resilient bodies than one might think.

Another example is the aforementioned geodesic dome developed by Buckminster Fuller (see Figure 2.8). Technically based on a series of 20 triangles with a framework of rigid struts capable of withstanding both compression and tension, the struts of a geodesic dome are connected over the shortest distance possible. The struts, or compression members, also form triangular (and sometimes pentagonal and hexagonal) shapes. Each structural element is oriented in such a way that each "joint" of the structure is maintained in a fixed position and tension is evenly transmitted throughout the whole structure, increasing stability and resiliency. While technically not a "true" tensegrity, geodesic domes nonetheless get their resilience from tensegrity principles. Modern camping tents also employ this kind of design, which ensures the dome's overall stability. This is one type of tensegrity structure.

The second type harkens back to the purer form of the floating compression sculptures of Kenneth Snelson, where the structural members that can bear compression are separate and distinct from those that can bear tension.

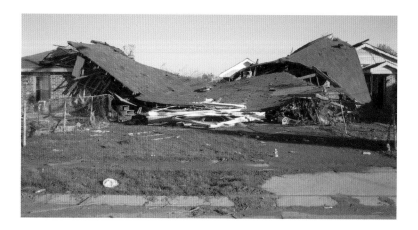

Figure 2.10

A caved-in house in New Orleans after Hurricane Katrina.

Courtesy of Infrogmation and Creative Commons. (https://creativecommons.org/licenses/by/2.5/deed.en)

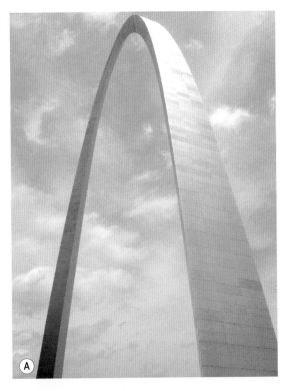
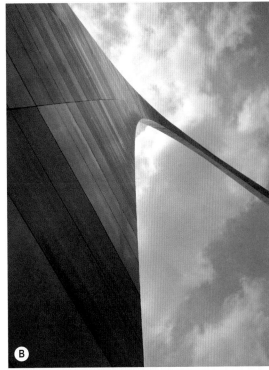

Figure 2.11
The Gateway Arch, St. Louis, Missouri.
Photos by author.

The balance of these forces creates a condition referred to as *prestress*. Prestress is the baseline tension inherent in a structure, or a body.

It is the prestress model that most closely reflects our own architecture, with the bones being the discontinuous, compression-bearing struts, and connective tissue being the cabling maintaining the tension. In fact, Dr. Levin found that bones *do not* fully compress with each other and their joint surfaces (Levin 1981) but rather our bones "float," if you will, like the rods in Snelson's sculptures, in the fascia and associated soft tissue.

The other crucial feature of either kind of tensegrity structure is that the tension is continuously transmitted throughout all the structural members. In other words, an increase of tension in one area would transmit that increase in tension throughout the whole. Likewise, a decrease in tension would ease the stress throughout the whole structure.

Let's try a thought experiment. Do you ever feel as if stress affects the tension level throughout your whole body? And once that stress is removed do you ever notice your entire body relax? Coincidence?

37

When referring to biological organisms, biotensegrity states that the body's 206 bones (compression struts) are being pulled up and held aloft against the force of gravity by the tensile force of fascia, ligaments, and tendons (tensional members). This truss-based design can be combined into ever-increasingly complex polygonal shapes that much better reflect our human architecture than the shapes of classical physics (Figure 2.12). But if you really want to see these ideas in action you should check the YouTube page of Boneman Pro. There you find mind-blowing videos of his fully articulated tensegrity skeletons.

Furthermore, given its recurrence in atoms of carbon, molecules of water, proteins, and cells, tensegrity is a basic principle of biological organization (Ingber 1998).

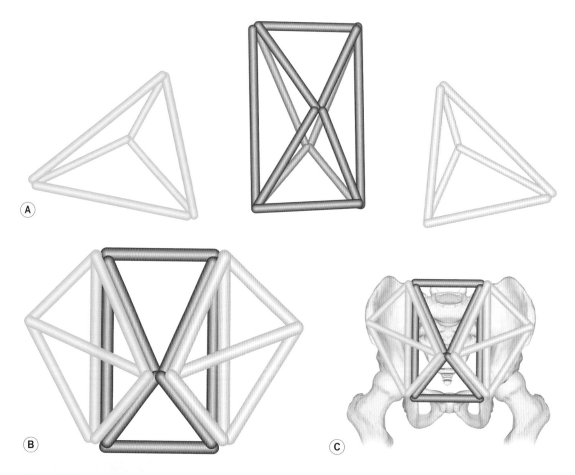

Figure 2.12

Four trusses or tetrahedrons (A). The middle one consists of two pentagonal trusses joined at the base. When joined together (B), they create shapes that much better approximate the shape of human architecture (C), in this case the hip.

Reproduced with kind permission from Carrie D. Gaynor and Jennifer Wideman.

Under the microscope

As a graduate student, cell biologist, and bioengineer, Donald Ingber was fascinated by how cells interacted mechanically. At the time cells were thought to be little more than amorphous water balloons, at least as far as their structure was concerned. It was during a 3D-modeling class that Ingber was exposed to early sculptures by Snelson and made a tensegrity sculpture himself out of sticks and strings (Ingber 1998). In so doing he noticed that the tensegrity sculpture behaved very much like a cell. When he pushed on it, it would spring back when the tension was released. When he pulled on it, it would warp and distort until the tension was released.

It was known that isolated cells behaved in mysterious ways when placed on different surfaces. For example, in a petri dish cells would spread out and flatten. When placed on flexible rubber, the cells would contract and become rounder and would also pull on and distort the rubber substrate (Harris et al. 1980). Note: the experiments were carried out on fibroblasts.

Using elastic string, wooden dowels, cloth, and wood, Ingber constructed a tensegrity-based model of a living cell (complete with a nucleus) and the underlying substrate. In short, he found that his model behaved very much like isolated cells. This model would eventually lead him to a series of experiments that would culminate with the publishing of his groundbreaking papers "Tensegrity I" and "Tensegrity II" (Ingber 2003a, 2003b).

Ingber embarked on a series of ingenious experiments that used magnetic beads and micropipettes to tug on the collagen cytoskeletons of the cells in order to change their shape. Simply put, he discovered that cells that were appropriately stretched thrived, whereas cells that became too rounded underwent apoptosis,

or cell death. By simply modifying the shapes of the cells, he and his team were actually able to change the cells' genetic programming.

At this point, it is best to quote the man himself:

Cells that spread flat became more likely to divide, whereas round cells that were prevented from spreading activated a death program known as apoptosis. When cells were neither too extended nor too retracted, they neither divided nor died. Instead they differentiated themselves in a tissue-specific manner: capillary cells formed hollow capillary tubes; liver cells secreted proteins that the liver normally supplies to the blood; and so on.

Thus mechanical restructuring of the cell and the cytoskeleton apparently tells the cell what to do. (Ingber 1998)

This is mechanotransduction at work (see Chapter 1). As a quick recap, the key player in mechanotransduction is integrin, which helps bind the cell to the extracellular matrix via the collagen matrix. When stimulated by pressure and vibration the integrin transmits that tension to the nucleus. This alters gene expression, affecting which genes switch on and off, and creates biochemical changes (see Figure 1.12). We still have so very much to learn about the process of mechanotransduction, and there is little doubt that many of our various manual therapies actually change genetic expression (Banes 2012).

But there is also tensegrity at work here, too, from the cellular level all the way up. Again, to quote Dr. Ingber:

From the molecules to the bones and muscles and tendons of the human body, tensegrity is clearly nature's preferred building system. Only tensegrity, for example, can explain how every time that you move your arm, your skin stretches, your extracellular matrix extends, your cells distort, and the interconnected molecules that form the internal framework of the cell feel the pull – all without breakage or discontinuity. (Ingber 1998)

From micro to macro

We can see the characteristic triangular patterns of tensegrity in the cytoskeleton of the cell (Figure 2.13) and it is now possible to see that even atoms themselves display a distinctive pattern of tensegrity (Figure 2.14). But does that scale up from micro to macro? How well does that actually translate to the entire human frame? Let's try a few simple experiments of our own to demonstrate how decreasing tension in one part of the body can remove strain from the rest of the body and, conversely, how specific stiffening of the tension (pre-tensioning) can create more stability in the body. You will feel it for yourself.

Let us start by removing some tension.

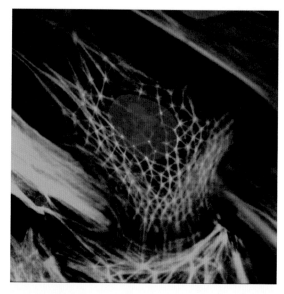

Figure 2.13
The actin monofilaments that comprise the cytoskeleton of a neonatal fibroblast.
Reproduced with kind permission from Professor Emilia Entcheva.

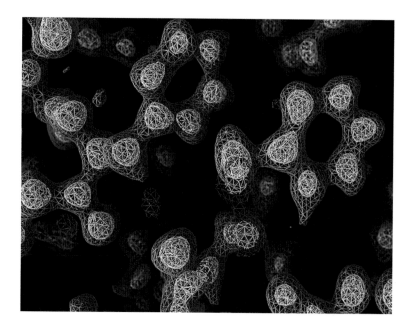

Figure 2.14
In 2020, atoms were visualized for the first time ever. Note the distinctive tensegrity in their fundamental structure.
Image courtesy of Paul Emsley and MRC Laboratory of Molecular Biology.

Experiment 1

This one may already be familiar to many of you, but I encourage all of you to try it.

1. Start by doing a simple standard forward bend.

   - Feel the strain, or lack thereof for you flexible folk, from the foot, through the back of calf up the hamstrings to the ischial tuberosities. Notice if one leg seems tighter than the other.

   - Next, carry that awareness into the back, and again differentiate between the two sides of your back, noticing where you feel tension.

   - Now, check in with your neck – is it tight or loose? Is your neck flexed? If so, let it relax and dangle, unless you are doing this in the jungle and have to watch out for predators!

   - Lastly, look at your hands. Notice how far they are from the ground or if one is lower than the other. Once you have a good sense of all those things, go back to standing.

2. Get a tennis ball, a small foam roller, or some other soft ball. No golf balls! Golf balls have no mercy.

   - Sit down, on the edge of a chair and place the ball or roller under one, and only one, bare foot.

   - Lean over the ball so that the loading pressure is exerted by the gravity of your slightly flexed torso and not by pushing down on it with your leg (Figure 2.15).

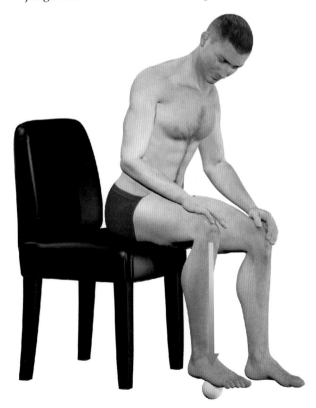

Figure 2.15
Experiment 1. The seated position for the exercise, leaning the torso over the leg and foot.

- Once you find the right amount of pressure, slowly, very slowly roll the ball back and forth along the plantar surface of your foot, from the tip of the heel to the ball of the foot (Figure 2.16). If you think you are going slowly enough, slow down even more. Do this for three to five minutes. This may seem like a long time, so I invite you to contemplate everything you have just read or listen to music or both.

3. Get up from the chair and compare the way your feet feel on the ground.

   - Now, repeat the forward bend. Is the tension the same on both sides? What do you feel in your back? Is one of your hands now lower than the other? How can this be?

   - Feel free to repeat this on the other foot before moving on.

   Now, let's increase stability.

Experiment 2

You will need a partner to do this one. And please make sure they have not recently injured their shoulder. It is all right – no-one will get hurt by this, but let's not aggravate an injury in the name of science if we can avoid it.

1. Stand perpendicular to your subject and have them hold their arm which is closest to you flexed to 90 degrees at the elbow joint.

2. Place your hands on the flexed arm and ask them to resist your pressure by flexing their arm muscles. Apply downward pressure and try to knock them off balance. It should be a relatively simple affair (Figure 2.17).

3. And for you Pilates folks who are reading this, try it again while engaging your core. It will help to stabilize you somewhat, but perhaps not as much as you might think.

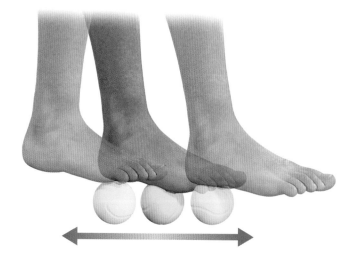

Figure 2.16
Slowly, very slowly, roll the ball along the area of the foot from the tip of the heel to the ball of the foot, stopping just short of the toes. Take your time, going slow enough to explore and release all the nooks and crannies.

4. Try this sequence again, but, this time, have your subject jam the tongue with great force into the roof of their mouth.

5. Apply downward pressure to the flexed arm.

Now, when you push down on the flexed arm you will find in almost all cases that the amount of force required to disrupt your subject's center of gravity has greatly increased, perhaps so much so that you will have to stop before you strain your wrist or injure the subject. And if they do that and activate their core, you have really lost.

How can this be?

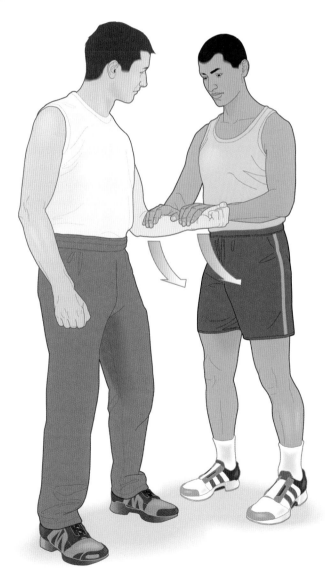

Figure 2.17
Experiment 2. Push down on the arm while pulling the arm toward you to disrupt their balance.

In Experiment 1 we are detensioning a tensegral fascial continuity known as the Superficial Back Line (see Figures 3.19 and 3.26). See Chapter 3 for more details.

In Experiment 2 we are increasing stability by pre-tensioning a fascial continuity and force transmission system known as the Superficial Back Arm Line (Figure 2.18), then deepening that stability by activating the Deep Front Line (Figure 2.19) – a fascial continuity that connects the muscle of the toes all the way up to the tongue.

In both exercises we altered the prestress of the body – in the first exercise by detensioning in order to relax the tissue and in the second by pre-tensioning to increase stability to perform an action (in this case not being knocked over). Pre-tension is a vitally important part of many physical activities, for example, accurately shooting a bow and arrow.

A further study of applying the principles of tensegrity to the human body was carried out in Poland, comparing changes in people with shoulder pain following treatment involving classic Swedish massage techniques where one group was treated with a standard approach and the other group was treated using the tensegrity model (Kassolik et al. 2013).

Applying very specific methodologies, for example, types of strokes, direction, duration, and so on, over a two-week period the control group received ten 20-minute massages of the shoulder region, specifically including the deltoid and glenohumeral joint.

The experimental group received the same number of massages in the same areas and of the same duration with one important difference: they were also evaluated and treated based on tensegrity principles. This meant that the areas treated included four additional regions, comprising 18 additional structures (Figure 2.20).

Subjects were palpated for tension along the "muscle–fascia–ligament system" in these areas and had additional Swedish-style treatments applied to them based on the palpatory findings.

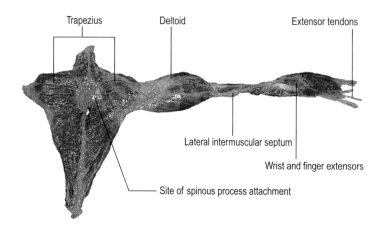

Trapezius Deltoid Extensor tendons

Lateral intermuscular septum

Wrist and finger extensors

Site of spinous process attachment

Figure 2.18
The Superficial Back Arm Line.
Photo by author. Reproduced with kind permission from Thomas W. Myers.

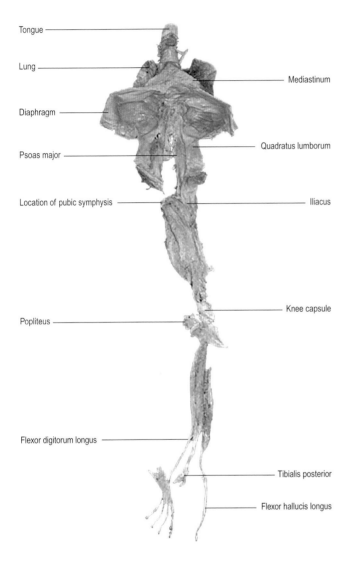

Tongue

Lung

Diaphragm

Psoas major

Location of pubic symphysis

Popliteus

Flexor digitorum longus

Mediastinum

Quadratus lumborum

Iliacus

Knee capsule

Tibialis posterior

Flexor hallucis longus

Figure 2.19
The Deep Front Line
Photo by author. Reproduced with kind permission from Thomas W. Myers.

The results were clear. While there were only 15 people in each group, a small number for this type of study, and both groups reported improvement in pain levels, the group that received massage based on tensegrity principles showed a statistically significant increase in both passive and active range of motion (ROM) during flexion and abduction.

Clearly, when it comes to tensegrity and the human body, it is time to rethink some of what we think we know about human anatomy.

LEFT		Testing locations	RIGHT	
DATE			DATE	

		Pathway for latissimus dorsi		
		External labium of iliac crest		
		Lateral edge of spinous process T5–7		
		Superior retinaculum for peroneal muscles		
		Pathway for pectoralis major		
		Crest of greater tubercle		
		ASIS (medial side)		
		Base of first metatarsal bone – peroneus longus		
		Pathway for serratus anterior		
		Superior angle of scapula		
		Coracoid process		
		Greater trochanter – superior and medial side		
		Inferior spinous fossa		
		Greater tubercle		
		Pathway for sacrotuberous ligament		
		PSIS		
		Sacrotuberous ligament		
		Central part of linea aspera		

Figure 2.20
Tensegrity approach. Patient's state evaluation card for the needs of massage based on tensegrity principle.
Reproduced from Kassolik et al. (2013) with permission from Elsevier.

References

Banes A J (2012) Mechanical loading & fascial changes – tendon focus. Plenary lecture, Third International Fascia Research Congress, Conference Proceedings DVD. Vancouver, BC: Canada.

Bartelink D L (1957) The role of abdominal pressure on the lumbar intervertebral discs. J Bone Joint Surg Br. November; 39-B (4) 718–725.

Biewener A A (1998) Muscle-tendon stresses and elastic energy storage during locomotion in the horse. Comp Biochem Physiol B Biochem Mol Biol. 120 (1) 73–87.

Borelli G A (1680) De Motu Animalium [On the Movement of Animals].

Choi C (2015) The Brontosaurus is back. Evolution blog, April 7. Available: www.scientificamerican.com/article/the-brontosaurus-is-back1 [May 18, 2022].

Försh P, Ólafson G, Carlsson T et al. (2016) A randomized, controlled trial of fusion surgery for lumbar spinal stenosis. N Engl J Med. April; 374 (15) 1413–1423.

Gatt R, Vella Wood M, Gatt A et al. (2015) Negative Poisson's ratios in tendons: An unexpected mechanical response. Acta Biomater. September; 24, 201–208.

Gracovetsky S (2008) The Spinal Engine, 2nd updated edn. p. 174 [Self-published].

Harris A K, Wild P and Stopak D (1980) Silicone rubber substrata: A new wrinkle in the study of cell locomotion. Science. April; 208 (4440) 177–179.

Ingber D E (1998) The Architecture of Life. Sci Am. January; 278 (1) 48–57.

Ingber D E (2003a) Tensegrity I. Cell structure and hierarchical systems biology. J Cell Sci. April; 116 (Pt 7) 1157–1173.

Ingber D E (2003b) Tensegrity II. How structural networks influence cellular information processing networks. J Cell Sci. April; 116 (Pt 8) 1397–1408.

Kassolik K, Andrzejewski W, Brzozowski M et al. (2013) Comparison of massage based on the tensegrity principle and classic massage in treating chronic shoulder pain. J Manipulative Physiol Ther. September; 36 (7) 418–427.

Kawakami Y, Muraoka T, Ito S et al. (2002) In vivo muscle fibre behaviour during counter-movement exercise in humans reveals a significant role for tendon elasticity. J Physiol. April; 540 (Pt 2) 635–646.

Levin S M (1981) The icosahedron as a biologic support system. Proceedings of the 34th Annual Conference on Engineering in Medicine and Biology. Houston, Texas, Volume 23, p. 404.

Levin S M (2011) The tensegrity-truss as a model for spine mechanics. J Mech Med Biol. 2 (3&4) 375–388.

Scarr G (2014) Biotensegrity: The Structural Basis of Life. Edinburgh, UK: Handspring Publishing, p. 34.

Snelson K (2013) Lecture appearance, Carnegie Museum of Art, Pittsburgh, Pennsylvania.

Further reading

Gracovetsky S (1988) The Spinal Engine. Vienna: Springer Verlag.

Lowell De Solórzano S (2021) Everything Moves: How Biotensegrity Informs Human Movement. Edinburgh, UK: Handspring Publishing.

Martin D-C (2016) Living Biotensegrity: Interplay of Tension and Compression in the Body. Munich, Germany: Kiener Press.

Scarr G (2014) Biotensegrity: The Structural Basis of Life. Edinburgh, UK: Handspring Publishing.

Fascia and Anatomy

3

No portion of the animal body has suffered so much at the hands of the descriptive anatomist as have those lowly tissues classed together as fascia. Whatever strides in the study of anatomy may be attributed to the introduction of formalin as a hardening and preservative reagent for anatomical material, it cannot be claimed that our conceptions, or our descriptions, of the arrangement of fascias have been made particularly clear by modern methods of practical anatomy.

For the medical student the study of the fascias of the body presents one of the most bewildering problems, and this is so partly because this tissue has remained undescribed in the types of lower animals he has dissected, and partly because in human anatomy the fascias are apt to be described without regard to their real significance and function. And yet fascia is of much interest for its own sake, and for the purpose of practical medicine and surgery few tissues so well repay the study devoted to them in practical anatomy.

—Frederic Wood Jones, 1920

Introduction

I will always remember teaching one of my first hands-on workshops in Columbus, Ohio. My teaching partner and I had been up all hours of the night before, making sure of the accuracy of every last detail. It was one of our first "solo" gigs, without the safety net of the older, wiser teacher to handle the hard questions. Of course, that also had a positive aspect – we would not be extra-nervous of failing in front of the older, wiser teacher.

There was, however, one student who was the current anatomy professor from a nearby college. He had held that post for almost two decades. He seemed the sort of person who would have been just as content to sit at home reading the research for the next three days, rather than attending the class. So, it was with the appropriate mix of confidence, bravado, and panic that I launched into the opening lecture.

About halfway through I presented some photographs from a preliminary (relatively crude) fascial dissection that another colleague and I had carried out on a continuity known as the Superficial Back Line (Figure 3.1). At this point the professor face-palmed, exclaiming painfully: "All these years and I've been throwing away the best part!"

This is par for the course in most first-year medical anatomy classes. Everything that is removed from the cadaver during dissection is scrupulously bagged and tagged so that it can be returned to the family for later interment, except, for the most part, the adipose tissue and the fascia, which is usually thrown into the garbage, although technically it is called "medical waste."

Even very detailed studies showing clear fascial connections between the iliac crest and lumbar vertebrae, separate from the lumbodorsal fascia (Bogduk 1980, Bogduk et al. 1982) do not make much impact. Fascia was further excluded even as recently as 2008, in a study of the iliotibial tract (ITT), more commonly referred to as the IT band (Benjamin et al. 2008). In an otherwise excellent dissertation on the ITT, Benjamin chose to follow the proposal of the Federative Committee on Anatomical Terminology to differentiate between fasciae and aponeuroses. In doing so, the decision was made to describe the tissue of the ITT as an aponeurosis (essentially, a broad, flat tendon) and remove anything that did not conform to that definition. In so doing, they excised one of the densest and most important portions of the ITT – the more ligamentous tissue that attaches to the lateral iliac crest (Figure 3.2).

This tissue, which is part of the fascia lata and the gluteal fascia, is vital in transmitting force from the knee to the hip (Figure 3.3) and also has implications as a tendon of insertion for the ITT (Stecco A. et al. 2013). This has also

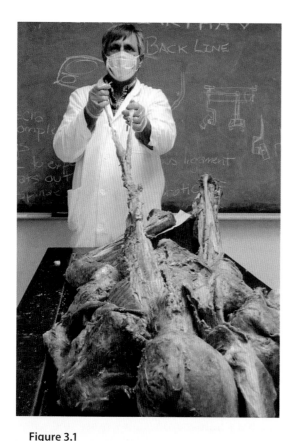

Figure 3.1
Initially, dissective explorations are not pretty. Here we see Tom Myers at the first exploration of the Anatomy Trains concept holding the hamstrings up and showing the fascial connections from the hamstrings to the sacrotuberous ligament and right on up to the erector spinae of the back. Dissection by author and Simone Lindner.
Reproduced with kind permission from Thomas W. Myers.

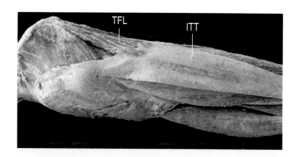

Figure 3.2
This dissection shows the fascia that comprises the iliotibial (IT) band (or iliotibial tract, ITT) primarily terminating at the tensor fascia lata (TFL).
Reprinted from Liem et al. (2017) with permission from Handspring Publishing.

On the surface it is easy to understand why the fascia continues to be disregarded. For one thing, it is in the way of the "good stuff" that the students most want, and indeed are trained to see. Also, anatomy books have largely omitted the fascia except where it is absolutely necessary (i.e., the plantar aponeurosis or the thoracolumbar fascia).

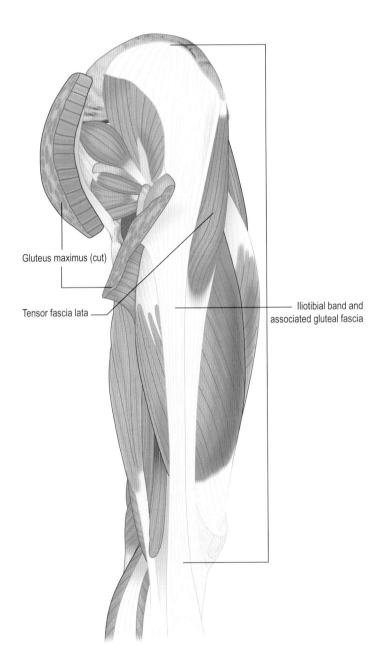

Gluteus maximus (cut)

Tensor fascia lata

Iliotibial band and
associated gluteal fascia

Figure 3.3
The upper leg, as it is more
conventionally illustrated, showing
the fascia of the iliotibial (IT) band
continuous with the iliac crest.
Note: the gluteus maximus has
been reflected, or pulled back,
to reveal the deep lateral rotators
beneath.

led some clinicians to recognize the probable
role of the gluteus maximus in both knee and IT
pain and treat accordingly. Yet this vital linkage
was excised in this otherwise excellent treatise
because it did not fit the distinct nomenclature,
although, to be fair, Benjamin has also published
papers that have helped to mainstream fascia
(Benjamin 2009).

Chapter Three

While I agree that embalmed cadaver fascia can appear as interesting as wet insulation, I do wonder if the very act of so very casually disregarding the connective tissue sets up an unconscious bias toward minimizing its importance? Does dissective exploration lead to dissective thinking?

In most of today's medical colleges, the gold standard textbooks for teaching anatomy are *Grant's Dissector* (Detton 2016), which provides step-by-step guidance on how to make everything look exactly as it is supposed to, and, with good reason, the anatomy atlas of Frank Netter (2014). Netter is an excellent and highly accurate reference. As a child, Netter longed to be a painter but instead enrolled in medical school and became a surgeon. Later he got to fuse his twin passions and is currently regarded as one of the finest medical illustrators ever.

Yet the joke, told to me by Tom Findley, co-founder of the Fascia Research Congress, goes like this:

What is fascia?

It's everything you don't see in Netter.

While one could argue that Netter did not have much use for fascia, it would be fairer to say that he did not have the training to understand the importance of everything he was seeing. This is a recurring theme in the history of anatomy.

In the beginning

Around 200 CE, the time of the Roman Empire and the great Greek physician and philosopher Galen, the idea of cutting up a human body to learn about its contents and how things might work was definitely anathema, if not downright sacrilegious. The early Christian Church forbade it, as did later the Catholic Church, and Islam.

So Galen learned anatomy (literal meaning, "to cut up" in Ancient Greek) by dissecting animals, predominantly pigs and monkeys. It was taken for granted that human anatomy was identical to the anatomy of these animals. So, of course, Galen got some things wrong, such as asserting the heart had three ventricles instead of four, and the liver had five lobes when it has none, but this tends to occur when assumptions collide at the intersection of discovery and learning.

These inaccuracies and outright wrong ideas, along with some correct ones, would continue to hold sway for approximately 1,100 years. Then in 1315, under Vatican sanction, the first recorded public human dissection took place in Bologna, Italy, under the guidance of Mondino de' Luzzi (Wilson 1987). His subsequent text, *Anathomia Mundini*, became the new standard on anatomy. Unfortunately, in a classic case of humans seeing exactly what they expect to see, it perpetuated all the inaccurate anatomical suppositions of Galen.

When Pope Sixtus IV decreed in 1482 that human dissection was permitted as long as the body was that of a convicted criminal and was later given a proper Christian burial, the study of human anatomy via cadaver dissection began to grow. Unfortunately, it was guided by the error-prone texts of de' Luzzi.

It is also important to note that during this time the prevailing attitude among physicians toward studying anatomy was one of mild disdain. Why get one's hands dirty and bloody when one could learn perfectly well everything one needed to know by reading the works of Galen and de' Luzzi? Besides, such work was for surgeons, who were regarded by physicians as little better than butchers at worst or highly skilled carpenters at best. And it was the physicians who controlled the medical colleges of the time. These prejudices would continue for another 75 years.

To comprehend more fully the state of anatomical study back then, imagine reading the works of the aforementioned anatomy experts without the benefit of accompanying illustrations. It seems downright ridiculous, but that is how it was in that era.

During the Middle Ages neither physicians nor artists were terribly interested in accurate depictions of the human body. This would change during the Renaissance when artists taught themselves to portray the body in realistic ways. Culturally, or at least among the monoculture of physicians and medical professors, there was a strong belief that illustrations would cheapen the subject. Medicine was serious business, not the stuff of books for children.

The first book to attempt to depict realistic drawings of human anatomy (key word here is "attempt") was the *Fasciculus Medicinae* [*Bundle of Medicine*] published in Venice in 1491. A collection of six different treatises from the late Middle Ages, it is perhaps best known for the somewhat notorious illustration of the "Wound Man" (Figure 3.4). While a groundbreaking book for its use of drawings, I wonder if illustrations like this reinforced the bias against their use in professional texts.

Ironically, or perhaps karmically, it was a doctor of medicine from Padua, Italy who would realize the full potential of medical illustrations. In so doing, he would revolutionize the study of medicine.

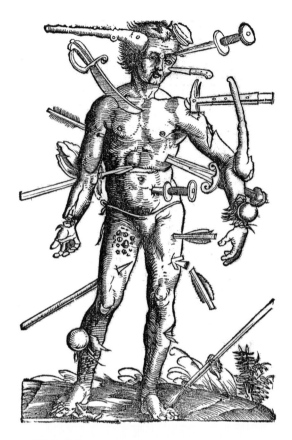

Figure 3.4
The infamous "Wound Man." Originating in 1491, these somewhat lurid and ridiculous drawings depicted the various wounds one might suffer from accidents or in battle. The accompanying text would suggest treatment options. This depiction, from 1519, includes a cannon ball.
Modified from Hans von Gersdorff. Courtesy of Wellcome Images.

A man from Padua

The story goes that when Andreas Vesalius (Figure 3.5) was teaching a class on the finer points of bloodletting (to reduce inflammation) he thought it might help clarify his teaching to prepare a large diagram of the veins of the body.

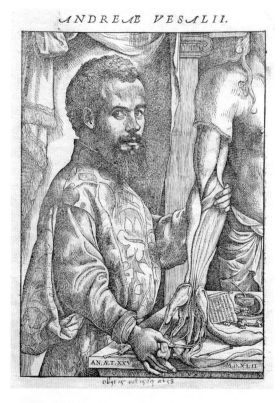

Figure 3.5

A portrait of Andreas Vesalius, father of modern anatomy.

copies are known still to exist. One might also say Vesalius invented niche publishing.

While popular, they were also inaccurate. In short, the *Tabulae* were right where Galen was right, and wrong where Galen was wrong. While they did include the five-lobed liver of Galen, Vesalius also thought to include an inset drawing of the liver that more accurately reflects what is known today. From this one could surmise that Vesalius's way of seeing was beginning to change.

Change came further still when Giunta Press decided to publish new editions of Galen's books in Latin and hired Vesalius to correct the existing translations. Work on the first few volumes was easy, but the third volume, *On Anatomical Procedures*, was so heavily revised that the managing editor at Giunta called it a virtual rewrite.

Six years later, in 1543, Vesalius's magnum opus *De Humani Corporis Fabrica* [*The Fabric of the Human Body*] was published. Meticulously detailed, annotated, and full of large, detailed illustrations that are considered to be from some of the finest woodcarvings of the sixteenth century, *De Humani Corporis Fabrica* set a new standard. While there was still much it got wrong (remember, preservatives and fixatives did not exist yet; and the rapidity with which bodies decay was the enemy of many an early anatomist), there was much more that it got right. It boldly threw out Galen's incorrect imaginings and in doing so insisted that the only way to understand the natural world was by observing and accurately, or as accurately as possible, documenting that world. While Vesalius did not invent the scientific method, he most certainly would have approved of it.

This went over so well with his students that Vesalius continued to produce more drawings to aid his lectures. One could say he invented PowerPoint.

It also helped that both Vesalius and the illustrators he employed were excellent at their craft (Figure 3.6). In 1538, Vesalius published six of his drawings. While not formally titled, they became collectively known as *Tabulae anatomicae sex* [*Six anatomic figures*]. Apparently, they were so popular and well used that only two complete

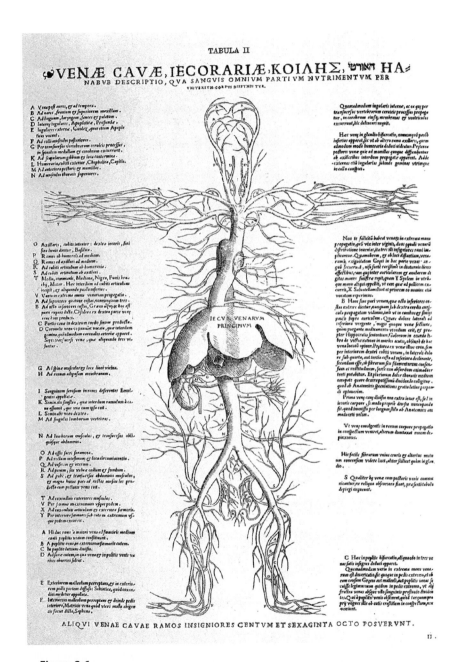

Figure 3.6

One of the first illustrations by Vesalius depicting the vena cava, liver, and distribution of the larger veins. From *Tabulae anatomicae sex* [*Six anatomic figures*].

Courtesy of Wellcome Library, London.

There are no great depictions of fascia in *De Humani Corporis Fabrica*, although there are plates that suggest connective tissue, alluding to potential patterns of force transmission (Figure 3.7).

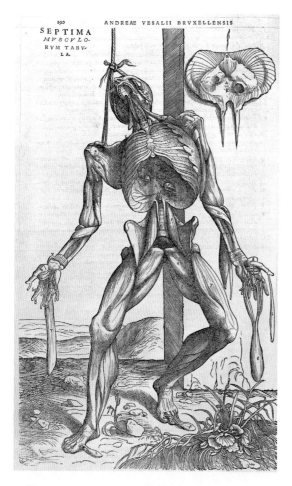

Figure 3.7

Plate from *De Humani Corporis Fabrica* by Vesalius. While again there is no depiction of fascia, the heavier black line going from the bottom of the foot and up the inside of the lower leg to the upper thigh and psoas does suggest a continuity (which we will see later in the Deep Front Line in Figure 3.23).

Courtesy of Wellcome Library, London.

This could be confirmation bias on my part but some have argued, given Vesalius's passion for accurate depiction of observations, that the inclusion of the heavier black lines appears to point to some kind of continuity. Certainly, that concept was there a little more than 150 years later, as can be seen in this passage from 1707 that connotes the necessity of healthy fascia in smooth, graceful movement:

The Use of the Membranes is, to wrap up and cover the Parts, to strengthen 'em, to defend several of them from being hurt by the subjacent Bones, to sustain the Vessels that are ramified upon them...

And while this solidifies fascia's reputation as a wrapping material, the passage continues:

...to keep the Parts united; and tis worth our Observation, that the admirable Sympathy, or consent of the Parts one with another, depends in a great measure upon their Fibrous Connexions. (Douglas 1707)

However, it would seem that the concept of fascia as an insulating layer or packing organ would only be solidified by the late 1800s, as can be seen by comparing these two passages:

Fascia (fascia, a bandage) is the name assigned to fibrous laminae of various extent and thickness, which are distributed through the different regions of the body, for the purpose of investing or protecting the softer and more delicate organs. (Wilson 1892)

and:

The fasciae (fascia, a bandage) are fibro-areolar or aponeurotic laminae of variable thickness and strength, found in all regions of the body, investing the softer and more delicate organs. (Gray 1893)

While both Wilson and Gray's seminal anatomy texts write about fascia within the context of muscles (and Gray does an admirable job writing about topological variations within the fascia), the above excerpts are as exciting as it gets for fascia at the turn of the nineteenth century. However, a quiet revolution was beginning "across the pond" (Gray and Wilson were both English).

The man from Kansas

Dr. Andrew Taylor Still (Figure 3.8), the founder of osteopathy, was born in 1828. One of nine children, his father was a medical doctor and a Methodist minister. When he was ten years old and suffering from a migraine headache, he would think to hang a loop of rope about eight inches from the ground and cushion the loop with a blanket. From there he rested the back of his head on the blanket, along the occipital ridge, and fell asleep. When he woke both headache and nausea had vanished. He would continue to repeat this self-treatment anytime he felt a headache coming on. Many years later he would realize that he had tractioned the occipital nerves and used a form of ischemic pressure to alter blood flow. By Still's later reckoning, it was the world's first osteopathic treatment.

In his early twenties he served a two-year apprenticeship with his father to learn to become a medical doctor. He also had a number of other occupations including farmer and school teacher. His fascination with engineering would lead him to patent a design for an improved butter churn and, much later in life, patent a smokeless indoor furnace. A staunch abolitionist, he was elected to the Kansas state legislature in 1857.

In 1861, at the age of 33, he enlisted in the Union Army during America's Civil War, serving in the infantry. While some sources have him serving

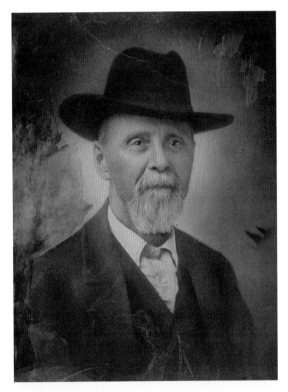

Figure 3.8
A portrait of Andrew Taylor Still, founder of osteopathy.
Museum of Osteopathic Medicine, Kirksville, Missouri
[1980.406.01].

as a hospital steward and performing surgeries, his autobiography mentions none of this; he was a soldier. In 1864, Andrew returned home from the war. Rather than finding respite upon reuniting with his family he found only sorrow. Three of his children died from spinal meningitis over a two-week period. Two weeks after that, his youngest daughter died of pneumonia.

While he fell into a deep grief, these events also sent him on the course that would change the way he practiced medicine. He endured new challenges and struggles, including being formally removed from the Methodist church for having the temerity to imitate Jesus by the "laying on of hands" to help cure sick people. Labeled an agent of Satan, he eventually relocated his family and practice to Kirksville, Missouri.

Andrew now referred to himself as a "lightning bone setter," but as his practice grew more successful he later coined the term "osteopath," eventually opening the American School of Osteopathy in 1892. One of the cornerstones of osteopathy is that the musculoskeletal system plays a vital role in both health and disease. He was especially fascinated by fascia.

In 1899, Dr. Still wrote that fascia:

...belts each muscle, vein, nerve, and all organs of the body. It is almost a network of nerves, cells and tubes, running to and from it; it is crossed and filled with, no doubt, millions of nerve centers and fibers to carry the work of secreting and excreting fluid vital and destructive. By its action we live, and by its failure we shrink, or swell, and die.

Furthermore:

Each fiber of all muscles owes its pliability to that yielding septum-washer, that gives all muscles help to glide over and around all adjacent muscles and ligaments, without friction or jar...It penetrates even its own finest fibers to supply and assist its gliding elasticity.(Still 1899)

Let's see just how far down those fibers go.

The "fasciomusculoskeletal" system

I am not advocating an even more complicated nomenclature, merely pointing out that even the common terminology "musculoskeletal" leaves out an essential component of how that system works. As mentioned earlier in this chapter, most anatomy books routinely skip the fascia in their renderings except when absolutely necessary. The fascial structures that are regularly included (the plantar fascia, iliotibial tract, thoracolumbar fascia, etc.) can also serve to reinforce the parts-based mentality. For example, the common portrayal of the upper leg looks something like Figure 3.9A in almost every anatomy book, yet the more fascially accurate version of the same thing would look something like Figure 3.9B. All the parts are still discernible, but there is the added layer of connectivity.

It is this layer, the deep fascia (sometimes referred to as the fascia profunda), that will be examined more closely in this chapter. Keep in mind that while this chapter will highlight layers and sublayers of the deep fascia, the fasciae at large form a single, unitary tissue that is no less divisible than the nervous or circulatory system.

The deep fascia

Unlike the loose connective tissue layer of fascia directly underneath the skin, the deep fascia is denser and much more highly organized than its superficial counterpart. Deep fascia contains all the layers that interact with the muscles (Figure 3.10) and as such includes all of the aponeurosis and the epimysial fascia (Stecco C. 2015).

The deep fascia is most easily thought of as a fibrous and elastic bodystocking or wetsuit. The innermost portion of this bodystocking peels away to form the epimysium, or a fascial pocket for each muscle. That is equivalent to about 640 pockets keeping each muscle separate yet connected. The orange analogy, albeit overused,

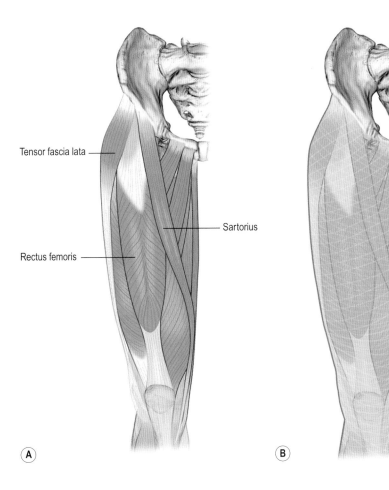

Tensor fascia lata

Sartorius

Rectus femoris

(A)

(B)

Figure 3.9
(A) The upper leg as typically presented.
(B) A depiction of the same leg in context with the epimysium or the "bodystocking" fascial layer.

is overused because it is the most succinct way to understand this concept (Figure 3.11).

The epimysium is also the layer that is continuous with the tendons that attach the muscles to the bones. These interconnected muscles, or myofascial units, are free to glide with respect to each other in their epimysial "pockets" due to a lubricating, hyaluronan-rich layer of loose connective tissue between them (Stecco C. et al. 2011). The epimysium is also implicit in epimuscular force transmission (Huijing 2007). It should also

be noted that there is a high density of contractile myofibroblasts in the perimysium (Borg & Caulfield 1980).

Related to the epimysium, and considered separate in form but not continuity, are the intermuscular septa. These tough, fascial sheets form discrete compartments or septums in the extremities (Figure 3.12). This arrangement of synergistic muscles packed into pressurized compartments increases the contractile efficiency of the muscles (Purslow 2010).

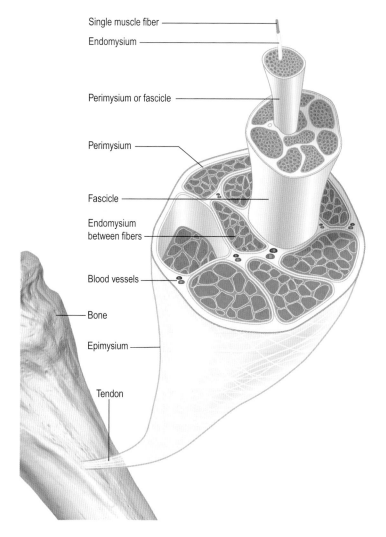

Single muscle fiber

Endomysium

Perimysium or fascicle

Perimysium

Fascicle

Endomysium
between fibers

Blood vessels

Bone

Epimysium

Tendon

Figure 3.10
The layers of the deep fascia from the epimysium of the muscle to the endomysium, which is the fascial wrapping of each muscle fiber.

Within the epimysium itself there is another layer of fascia called the perimysium (Figure 3.13). The perimysium wraps groups of muscle fibers into smaller bundles. These smaller bundles are also sometimes referred to as "fascicles," although the term "fascicle" can be ascribed to any "bundle" of structures (such as nerve fibers). While ostensibly a series of smaller pockets, the perimysium runs in

continuity with the epimysium at the exterior of the muscle.

Still the fascia does not stop there. Each muscle fiber, or myofiber, is wrapped in a tunic of fascia called endomysium (Figure 3.14). The endomysium forms a continuous lattice, connecting all the muscle fibers within the perimysium. This honeycomb of collagen enables load sharing

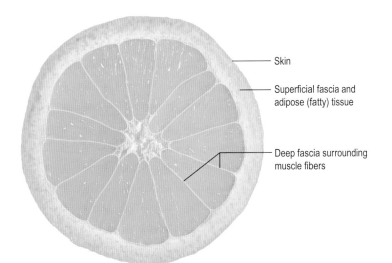

Skin

Superficial fascia and adipose (fatty) tissue

Deep fascia surrounding muscle fibers

Figure 3.11
The classic orange model –
a good example of how the
superficial fascia and the deeper
epimysial layer form one tissue
that both interconnects and
separates the inner contents.

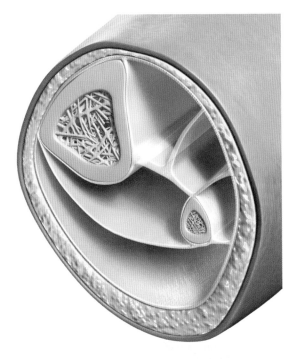

Figure 3.12
The fascial compartments of the lower leg.
Illustration courtesy of fascialnet.com.

among the individual myofibers, forming yet another kind of biotensegrity. But again, the fascia does not stop there.

Going back to the electron microscope, it can also be seen that collagen fibers create a longitudinal network (Figure 3.15), right through the epimysium to the adjacent, antagonistic muscle. And it does not stop there either. Going in closer, the collagen fibers continue to divide smaller and smaller, going all the way down to the level of the cell membrane (Figure 3.16A and B).

So, what we have is a fibrous network, a single continuity within the body from the undersurface of the skin, all the way down to the nucleus of the cell. These fibers connect the inside of the cell to the outside of the cell and its immediate environment forming a body-wide network that responds to force and tension.

If the fascial system is that vast and complex, how can it be simplified in order to better understand it in an anatomical context? Perhaps by creating some good maps.

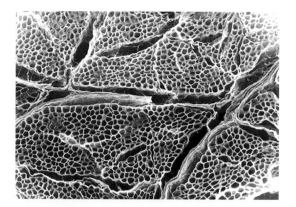

Figure 3.13

Electron microscope image of the perimysium and endomysium in a piece of beef. The smaller tubes indicate the endomysium and the bigger and broader pieces of collagen indicate the perimysium.

Reprinted by permission of Springer Nature from the *Journal of Muscle Research and Cell Motility*. The morphology and mechanical properties of endomysium in series-fibred muscles; variations with muscle length. Purslow, P.P., Trotter, J.A., 15 (3) 299–304. 1994.

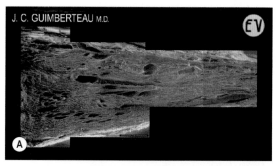

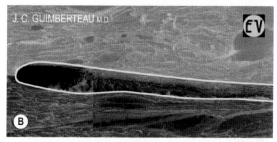

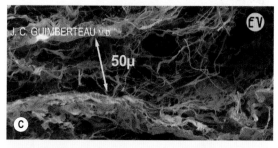

Figure 3.15

(A) The longitudinal collagenous network between the tibialis and gastrocnemius in a rat. (B) A close-up highlighting the area of "separation" between the two muscles. (C) A further close-up, 50 microns in length (approximately 0.0019685 of an inch), of the same area.

From "Muscle Attitudes" DVD. Reproduced with the kind permission of Endovivo Productions and J.-C. Guimberteau MD.

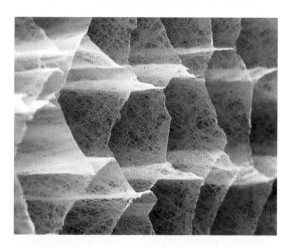

Figure 3.14

Extreme detail shot of the individual endomysial tubes. Note the intertwined collagen network even at this level.

Reprinted by permission of Springer Nature from the *Journal of Muscle Research and Cell Motility*. The morphology and mechanical properties of endomysium in series-fibred muscles; variations with muscle length. Purslow, P.P., Trotter, J.A., 15 (3) 299–304. 1994.

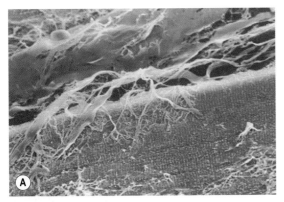

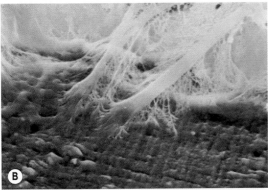

Figure 3.16
(A) Individual collagen fiber and scaffolding at the endomysial level via scanning electron micrograph. (B) This image shows the perimysium merging with endomysium.
Reprinted from Passerieux et al. (2006) with permission from Elsevier.

Yes, it is all connected

Frederic Wood Jones

Frederic Wood Jones was Professor of Anatomy at the University of Melbourne in Australia, and later became the Chair of Anatomy at the University of Manchester, in the United Kingdom. Widely published in a variety of topics and highly regarded, Wood Jones is perhaps most well known for staking a strong position against

Charles Darwin, considering the similarities between humans and apes to be an example of convergent evolution.

Convergent evolution theory posits the natural trend of widely divergent species to evolve similar traits. A common example would be the ability to fly. Mosquitoes, hummingbirds, and bats all share this ability, but do not share a common ancestor or even species. Wood Jones did not believe that man shared a common ancestor with primates and furthermore thought it ludicrous that man ever went through a brachiating, tree-swinging phase. If man did have a common mammalian ancestor, Wood Jones believed it would have been from the tarsier spectrum (Figure 3.17). His ability to think outside the box was definitely borne out in his views on human anatomy.

A lively and incisive writer, Wood Jones was not prone to dissective thinking. He challenged the orthodoxy of muscle origins and insertions, writing in 1920:

Movement is affected by the action of muscles working in groups... A muscle does not necessarily do in life what the dissected muscle, or a mechanical contrivance will do in a cadaver. Neglect of this fact has led to many errors in teaching. (Wood Jones 1920)

Wood Jones seemed to have had an excellent understanding of the functional importance of fascia, particularly the gliding qualities, but it was the differences in the fascia of the limbs that held his attention the most. In his view, the precision of the fascial septa and attachments in the arms stood in stark contrast to the fascial connections in the legs. He found the leg much harder to dissect because of how enmeshed the muscles are with the fascia. Many of the leg

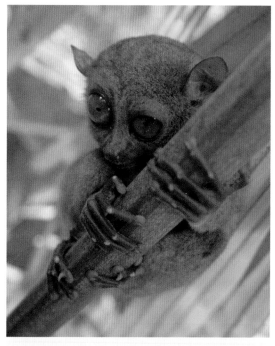

Figure 3.17
The tarsier. It was something about the similar dental structure that led Wood Jones to posit a similarity to *Homo sapiens*, not the exquisite shape of their hands.
Courtesy of Jasper Greek Golangco.

muscles end in broad fascial expansions and some, such as the tensor fascia latae, attach directly to the fascia. Not to mention the tougher septa that serve to compartmentalize the leg (see Figure 3.12).

To Wood Jones, the differences were of the "form follows function" variety – or perhaps "function creates form" is more accurate. To him, the greater preponderance of fascia in the leg indicated a dual function, with the fascial structure of legs indicating both the need for strong but essentially passive postural support as in standing, and also movement, and powerful movement when needed, as in locomotion.

Overall, Wood Jones likened the fascial net to an exoskeleton within the arm and legs. This image also brings to mind Andry Vleeming's lovely metaphor of fascia being the "soft skeleton" of the body.

Kurt Tittel

Author of more than 500 scientific papers and a handful of books considered classics in the field, Dr. Kurt Tittel is regarded by many as one of the fathers of sports medicine in Germany. Former Professor Emeritus of the Department of Functional Anatomy of the University of Halle in Germany, Dr. Tittel believed that to base the study of anatomy solely on dead material (dissection) was too limiting. Instead, he advocated a study of anatomy that was "focused on life, on active functioning which is oriented toward practical needs."

Not unlike many somatic pioneers (see Chapter 8), Tittel saw structure and function as two sides of the same coin. No part, no one muscle or bone, could be adequately understood without taking into consideration its relationship to the whole organism. Quite presciently, Dr. Tittel believed that this relationship between structure and function was mirrored all the way down to the cellular level.

While Dr. Tittel understood the dynamic plasticity potential of soft tissue inherent in athletic training, his primary focus was on the muscles. His ideas were also applicable to the connective tissue sheaths and aponeurosis (fascia), but he did not dwell on the fasciae as such, nor did he recognize their full potential.

What his passion for functional anatomy and painstaking attention to detail have left is the concept of muscle slings. These functional slings are painstakingly detailed in his seminal work *Muscle Slings in Sport* (Figure 3.18). First published in 1956, it remains in print to this day.

While conceivably influenced by the German anatomist Hermann Hoepke and his *Das* *Muskelspiel des Menschen* (*The Muscleplay of Man*, 1936, out of print), Tittel's book presents more than three-dozen muscle slings and an unparalleled trove of ideas about movement, specifically sport-related movement, which continue to inspire and influence.

Subsequent decades would continue to see further concurrent developments along the

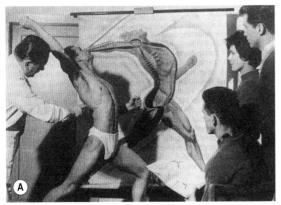

Figure 3.18
From initial modeling and drawing (A, B), to analysis and final rendering of the functional muscle slings (C), the painstaking work of Kurt Tittel.
Reproduced with kind permission from Christl Kiener Publishing.

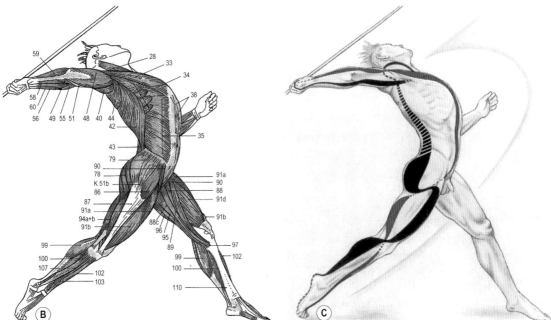

lines of the muscle-sling, and indeed fascial sling, theories. Two notable known examples would be Vladimir Janda's "Upper Crossed" and "Lower Crossed" models and the fascia chains of Serge Paoletti DO; however, to say these were directly influenced by Tittel would be at best speculative and at worst completely false.

Perhaps we could ascribe these, and the next example, to academic convergent evolution.

Thomas Myers

Thomas Myers was a practitioner of Rolfing® Structural Integration, a type of fascial body-work. As developed by Ida P. Rolf (see Chapter 8), Rolfing® revolved around the recipe of a fixed number of treatments that, while individually tailored, were nonetheless delivered in a very specific order. Myers was impressed with how well the system worked for most people. He was equally obsessed with finding out the underlying anatomical reasons as to why this would be so.

He was in a unique position to do it, too, serving as both an anatomy teacher at the Rolf Institute® in Boulder, Colorado, and also teaching pretrainings for the European Rolf Institute® in Germany from 1981 into the 1990s.

Oddly enough, for all the time spent teaching in Germany over the years, Myers would not be exposed to any of the muscle slings of Tittel or Hoepke. Myers was, however, familiar with Australian anatomist Raymond Dart's ideas from his studies of the Feldenkrais method of somatic education. While Dart's theory of the double spiral would certainly influence Myers, at the time that was all he knew of other notions of interconnected anatomy.

The groundwork that led to the development of his Anatomy Trains system of myofascial

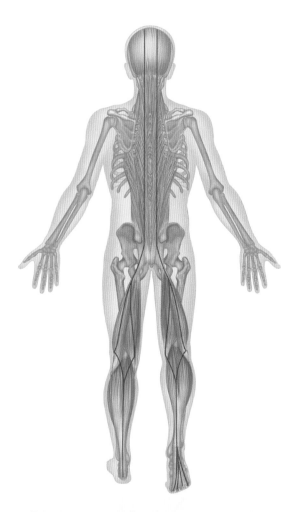

Figure 3.19
The Superficial Back Line, which is a fascial continuity that goes from the plantar fascia, calcaneal periosteum and up the back of the legs to the erector spinae, via the sacrotuberous ligament, and up the neck to the galea aponeurotica.

meridians happened during these years and started as a classroom game. Myers despaired of teaching a dry anatomy class, following the rote method of origin, insertion, innervation,

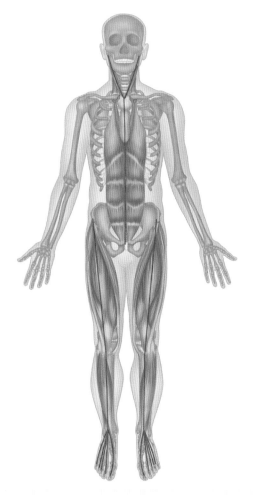

Figure 3.20
The Superficial Front Line, which covers the anterior surface of the body with a mechanical connection at the hip to connect the upper and lower aspects in flexion and extension only.

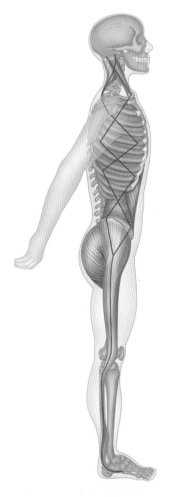

Figure 3.21
The Lateral Line, which governs both stability and mobility, as well as lateral flexion and extension.

and so on. To his mind such a traditional method may get the job done but rarely leaves a lasting impression.

More importantly, he wanted to share his passion and impart a true working knowledge of anatomy in the minds of students.

Inspired by the systems-based thinking of one of his former professors, Buckminster Fuller, he created a game of "What does this part connect to?" He theorized that connecting the parts to larger wholes would make everything more memorable. This approach exceeded his wildest dreams.

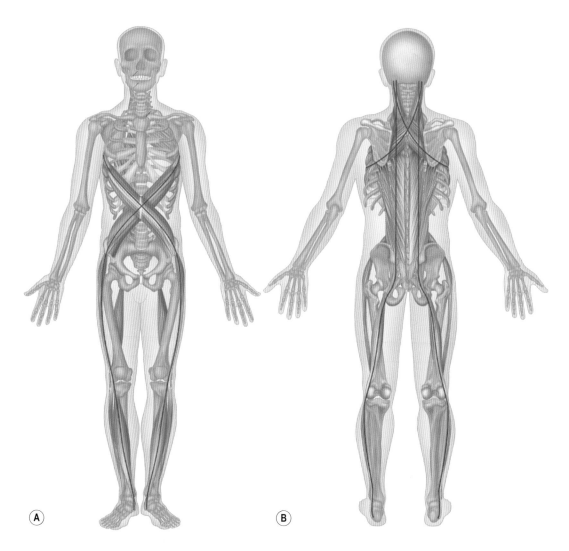

Figure 3.22
Winding its way through the previous three superficial lines is the Spiral Line, which creates and transmits spiral and oblique forces through the body.

While it would take years for the emerging patterns to come to full fruition, Myers would publish his first papers on the Anatomy Trains model in 1997. The subsequent book, *Anatomy Trains*, would be first published in 2001, go through four editions, and be translated into 13 languages.

The Anatomy Trains model presents the anatomy of connection via a series of 13 whole-body myofascial maps that conform to both patterns of

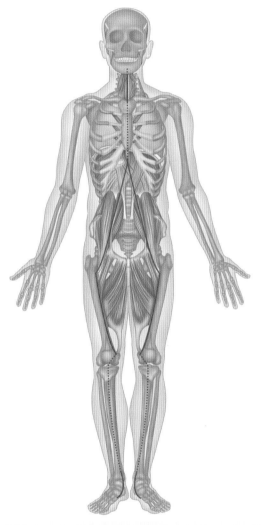

Figure 3.23
The inner core of our body, the Deep Front Line, which is also an interface between the musculoskeletal and visceral body.

The Anatomy Trains are organized around lines (see Figures 3.19–3.25). Three of these lines go from head to toe and cover the more superficial aspects of the dorsal, ventral, and lateral aspects of the body (Figures 3.19–3.21). In the transverse plane, the spiral line covers the myofascial linkages involving spiral and rotational movements (Figure 3.22). In the core there is the Deep Front Line that includes fascial aspects of the viscera and also has a more volumetric aspect (Figure 3.23).

There are four lines for the arm (Figure 3.24 A–D) and lastly, three functional lines, named for their specificity in functional movement (Figure 3.25). (Note: The third functional line, the Ipsilateral Functional Line, is a relatively recent finding and is not covered here.)

It is all well and good, and probably true, to say, "It's all connected," but it is not especially helpful. The Anatomy Trains model presents a coherent scheme that shows the clinician, therapist, or anyone involved in biomechanics exactly how everything is connected and the clinical relevancies.

A good example of the Anatomy Trains continuity model is the Superficial Back Line (SBL) that connects the plantar fascia to the periosteum of the calcaneus, up the Achilles tendon to the gastrocnemius, which has crosslinks with the descending hamstrings. The fascia on the hamstrings is contiguous with the sacrotuberous ligament that then expands into the erector spinae up the length of the back to the galea aponeurotica (Figure 3.26AB). This continuous myofascial chain has withstood the test of multiple embalmed and fresh fascial dissections. Not every Anatomy Trains line has withstood this scrutiny.

myofascial force transmission and the principles of biotensegrity. They also conform to a specific set of internal rules. There are a few exceptions where the rules are modified and, when they are, it is done both intelligently and plausibly.

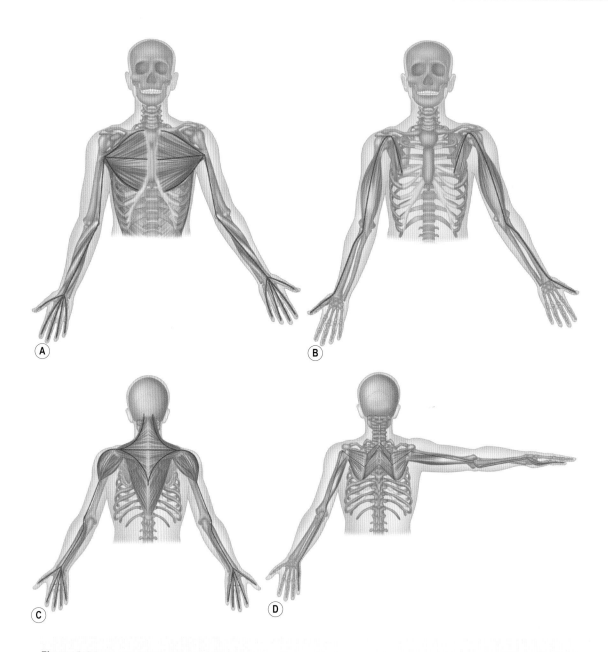

Figure 3.24
(A) The Superficial Front Arm Line (SFAL), which connects the pectoralis major to the fingers. (B) Underlying, assisting, and stabilizing the SFAL is the Deep Front Arm Line, often an area of fascial restriction in our digital age. (C) The Superficial Back Arm Line, which coordinates movement in the arm and shoulder posteriorly and laterally. (D) The Deep Back Arm Line, which also includes the muscles of the rotator cuff.

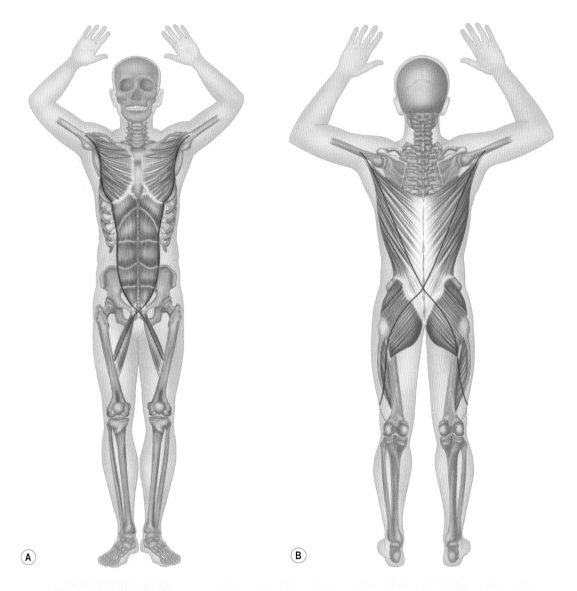

(A) (B)

Figure 3.25
The Front Functional Line (A) and the Back Functional Line (B) serve to leverage force transmission through the arms via the trunk and legs and vice versa.
Figures 3.19–3.25 are reproduced with kind permission from Thomas W. Myers and Lotus Publishing.

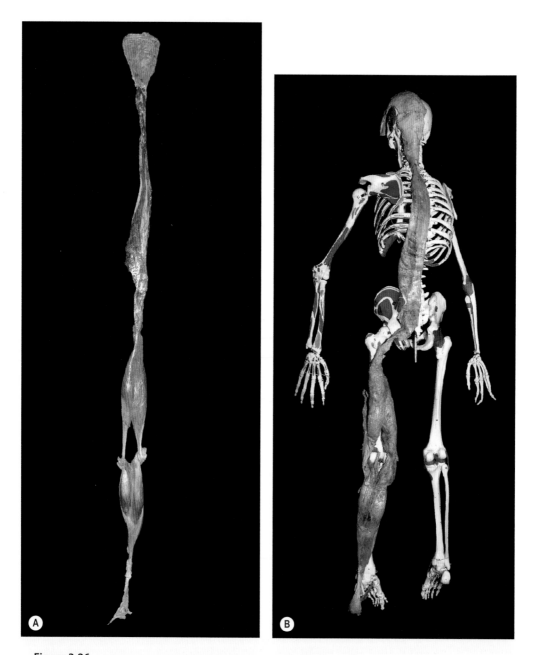

Figure 3.26
Two dissected views of the Superficial Back Line. (A) A specimen from a fresh cadaver.
(B) An embalmed specimen overlaid onto a skeleton to add dimensionality.
Reproduced with kind permission from Thomas W. Myers.

Full disclosure: I have been involved behind the scalpel, behind video and still cameras, documenting many of these dissections. I also had the distinct honor and embarrassment to have been the first person to shred through a sternalis on the Superficial Front Line. Even though one exploration does not a map make, it seemed obvious to all that the relative flimsiness of such a structure called into question the nature of the upper Superficial Front Line.

A systematic review of peer-reviewed anatomical dissection studies looked for independent evidence for the existence of six of the 13 myofascial meridians (Wilke et al. 2016). The team did this by looking for evidence of continuity in the transition points of lines. The results suggested strong evidence for the reality of the SBL (based on 14 studies), the Back Functional Line (eight studies), and the Front Functional Line (six studies). The Lateral Line, Spiral Line, and Superficial Front Line did not fare so well. Although the study concluded that just because researchers could only verify about half of the transition points for both the Lateral and Spiral Lines, this did not negate their possible existence as myofascial continuities. It is also of note that the SBL has withstood extensive electromyographic testing (Weisman et al. 2014). This is one myofascial continuity that objectively seems to be on very solid footing.

While the Anatomy Trains are excellent maps for understanding whole-body, holistic functional anatomy, as well as force transmission and repetitive strain or trauma-based compensation patterns, it would be silly to think: "That's it! We've found all the connections."

There are many other fascial connections being discovered.

Other vital connections

Ligaments, dynaments, and the new order

The research of Jaap van der Wal (2009) furthered the "It's all connected" idea by showing how muscle and joint connective tissue are part of a continuum running in series with each other rather than in parallel. Using fascia-sparing dissective techniques, van der Wal threw cold water on the accepted belief that ligaments are deep to the muscle tendon and that they are only active during the end ranges of joint movement. Instead, he found specialized connective tissue structures organized in series with muscle fascicles. Specific collagen fibers running between the bones are a rare occurrence. Instead, perimysial muscle fascicles insert directly into the broader, more aponeurotic fascia of the epimysium that then attach to the periosteum of the bone (Figure 3.27AB). Van der Wal considers this arrangement to be "dynamic ligaments" or "dynaments."

Taken together, the dynaments form a continuous complex that adjusts its overall length based on how a person is moving. As Tom Findley elegantly summarized:

There are only two places in the body where the bones don't change distance when they move: the knee joint and C1-C2. Everywhere else, when I move my muscle, the tendon has to get shorter on the flexed side and longer on the extended side. According to van der Wal, there is "no functional difference between a muscle and a ligament." (Findley 2013)

Indeed, van der Wal considers ligaments to be largely artifacts of the dissector's scalpel.

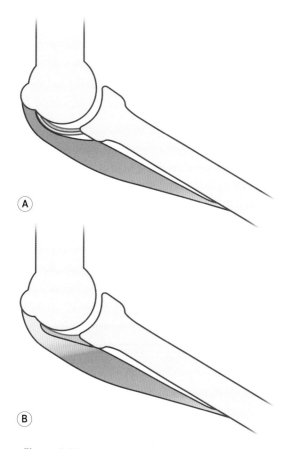

(A)

(B)

Figure 3.27

(A) The classic parallel anatomical view of the muscle, tendon, and ligament as separate structures. (B) van der Wal's dynament model where the muscle, tendon, and ligament are in series as part of the same continuum of tissue.

Adapted with kind permission from Jaap van der Wal.

The new "low back"

Since the 1990s Belgian researcher Andry Vleeming and American Frank Willard have been exhaustively studying that diamond of white that appears in every anatomy text – the thoracolumbar fascia or TLF (Willard et al. 2012). A crucial structure of the low back,

the TLF comprises three separate but connected layers approximately 5.5 mm thick on average. The outermost layer has more parallel collagen fibers in a thin sheet that run perpendicular to the spine, whereas the middle layer fibers run obliquely and are in thicker bundles, and the inner layer is loose connective tissue. The inner and outer layers also contain free nerve endings (Mense 2019) (see Chapter 4). The TLF is a crucial load-transfer point forming a crossover architecture from the upper limbs to the lower limbs. The forces from loads actually transmit diagonally across the latissimus through to the gluteus on the opposite side (Vleeming et al. 1995). That reality furthers another interesting notion that the TLF can also serve to function like a tendon for the contralateral gluteus and thus becomes the prime driver in the spring-like gait of African swing walkers (Zorn & Hodeck 2011).

Structurally, the TLF forms a soft-tissue girdle or myofascial ring that posits itself between the bony rings of the hips and rib cage. One key feature of the TLF is the lumbar interfascial triangle (LIFT) (Schuenke et al. 2012). The LIFT is the interface between the abdominal muscles and the TLF. The common tendon of the transversus abdominis (the largest muscle in the body) splits along the posterior fascial envelope of the quadratus lumborum to join with the middle and posterior layer of the TLF, forming a triangular pocket (Figure 3.28). More than 800 MRIs were examined to verify the existence of this structure (Vleeming 2017).

The LIFT is a big reason why the torso is not ruptured when major forces are put through the body, such as in heavy lifting. Collectively, when all these muscles contract, force is transmitted not only longitudinally but also along all the

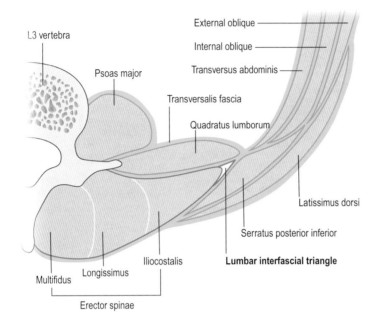

L3 vertebra

Psoas major

External oblique

Internal oblique

Transversus abdominis

Transversalis fascia

Quadratus lumborum

Latissimus dorsi

Serratus posterior inferior

Iliocostalis

Longissimus

Multifidus

Lumbar interfascial triangle

Erector spinae

Figure 3.28
The low back complex from a fascial perspective with the lumbar interfascial triangle (LIFT) as a point of convergence. The tendon of the transversus abdominis (which blends into the LIFT) is capable of tensing the posterior layer of the lumbodorsal fascia or PLF. The PLF is itself a fascial blending of the latissimus dorsi (at the most superficial level) as well as the multifidus, longissimus and the iliocostalis (contained within the paraspinal retinacular sheath). It can also include the serratus posterior inferior (SPI), although the fascia from the SPI is not usually present below the level of L3.
Reproduced from Willard et al. (2012) with permission from John Wiley & Sons.

parallel connections, including the dynaments, creating a hydraulic amplification (Figure 3.29) that serves to stabilize the entire vertebral column while creating 30 per cent more efficiency for the muscles (Hukins et al. 1990). It has also been shown that people with chronic low back pain exhibit 25 per cent greater thickness in the thoracolumbar fascia when compared to pain-free groups (Langevin et al. 2009). This thickness also coincides with changes in viscosity of hyaluronan, further compromising the gliding behaviors of the underlying fascial layers, contributing to the symptoms often identified as myofascial pain.

Metaphorically this suggests to me that the transversus abdominis "feeds" the TLF, and therefore the low back, like the river feeds the sea. Clinically, during therapeutic interventions, I find this very useful imagery for helping patients with low back pain to locate this area.

A woman in Padua

Carla Stecco started young. Her fascination with fascia began when, under the guidance of her father, physiotherapist Luigi Stecco (see Chapter 8), she dissected small animals to better understand the fascia (or, as game hunters call it, the "silver skin"). She became an orthopedic surgeon and spent considerable time in her mid-twenties at the University of Paris, where she honed her fresh-tissue dissection skills and further developed her theories about the role of fascia in the human body. As a perusal of the references in this volume will show, she, along with her MD brother Antonio Stecco, has been responsible for many groundbreaking discoveries in the field of fascia science.

Now, almost exactly 500 years after the birth of Vesalius, Carla is Professor of Human Anatomy and Movement Science at the University of Padua

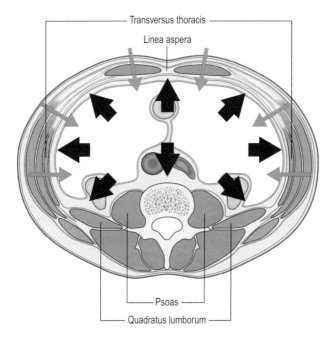

Transversus thoracis
Linea aspera
Psoas
Quadratus lumborum

Figure 3.29
Transverse section of the thorax. Force transmission occurs not just longitudinally but also in parallel connections as indicated by the arrows in this cross-section of the trunk. As muscles contract they tension parallel fibers to create an outward force and the surrounding tissue pushes back in. This is the foundation for abdominal bracing, which increases efficiency and speeds force transmission. As such this demonstrates how muscles can push as well as pull.
Adapted from Luchau (2016) with permission from Handspring Publishing.

(Figure 3.30). She has also published the first proper anatomical atlas of fascia (Stecco C. 2015). It should be noted that she performed all the dissections and took all of the photographs in this work. Taking a decade to produce, this book sets a new standard in the field. Professor Stecco's atlas also features ongoing sections highlighting the clinical relevancy of her anatomical and histological findings, no doubt another nod to the influence of her father, and this is deeply appreciated by this clinician and every therapist who approaches her work.

Professor Stecco's book serves to integrate the fascial and muscular systems in ways that no prior text has done, and with the thoroughness, accuracy, and attention to fine detail only found in the finest medical textbooks. For anyone working in the fascial field, this enlightening tome will keep you very, very busy in the best possible way.

Not one to rest on her laurels, Carla continues to break new ground with her research and also became one of the project directors in the most ambitious attempt yet to visualize the human fascial system.

The fascial net plastination project

A hundred and fifty kilometers southeast of Berlin, Germany, is the small town of Guben. Situated along the border with Poland, it is a divided city with its other half, Gubin, officially part of Poland since 1945. While this synthetic line, the Oder-Neisse Line, mostly follows the Oder and Lusatian Rivers the historical circumstances that bifurcated this town are quite arbitrary. Perhaps this makes Guben uniquely suited to bridge the somewhat arbitrary worlds of classical anatomy with fascial anatomy. Less metaphorically, Guben is home to the Plastinarium (Figure 3.31),

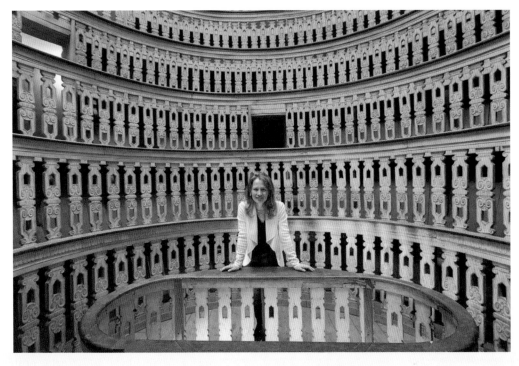

Figure 3.30
Carla Stecco in the Anatomy Theater at the University of Padua.

a museum, educational facility and producer of one-of-a-kind anatomical specimens to universities, medical universities, healthcare concerns, and, most famously, BODY WORLDS. Brainchild of Dr. Gunther von Hagens and CEO/Curator Dr. Angelina Whalley, and one of the most successful traveling exhibits on the planet, BODY WORLDS' mission to educate and inspire the general public about the inner workings and proper care of the human body has attracted more than 50 million visitors in over 140 cities since 1995.

While there is certainly fascia to be seen in many of the finished plastinates (the generic name for the finished pieces), there were no exhibit pieces specifically devoted to it – although over the years this idea had been suggested by many in the fascia

research community to those affiliated with BODY WORLDS. In August of 2017 this would change when Robert Schleip, researcher and co-founder of the International Fascia Congress, met with Plastinarium CEO Rurik von Hagens, and the Director of Anatomy and Plastination, Dr. Vladimir Chereminskiy. Robert's ambitious proposal was to assemble an ongoing team of volunteer dissectors from around the world to work with the Plastinarium to create three full-body fascial plastinates – one superficial, one deep, and one containing the deeper "core" and visceral fasciae.

To create a plastinate of any kind worthy for display is a painstaking five-step process. It starts with the initial dissection of a formalin-preserved specimen and then the piece (or whole body)

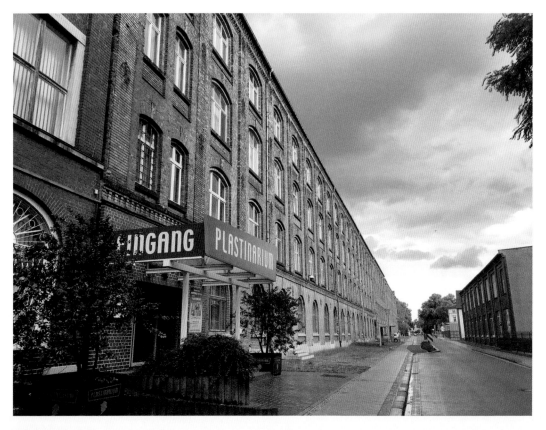

Figure 3.31

The immense Plastinarium in Guben, Germany.

Photo by Lauri Nemetz. Reproduced with permission from The Fascial Net Plastination Project, www.fasciaresearchsociety.org/plastination.

undergoes a dehydration and de-fatting process via a series of acetone baths. Once that is completed the specimen is submerged under vacuum pressure in a liquid polymer that infuses it in silicone rubber all the way down to the cellular level. So, for a full body from dissection through final "vacuum-sealing" it is a six-month process. Then the specimen is ready for final positioning. This is another elaborate process involving constant, small, careful adjustments to the plastinate (because rubber can rip). Additionally, metal rods, wire, blocks, mesh, and hundreds and sometimes thousands of pins are needed to hold everything exactly in place. Every bit of tissue, including nerves and blood vessels, must be accounted for and kept intact throughout this process. Once the final positioning has been approved by a panel from the Plastinarium (think the anatomical equivalent of Olympic judges) the plastinate is placed in an airtight container for a final gas-curing process, another step that can take days or weeks. Next, any remaining positioning tools are removed, colorization and touch ups performed, and the piece is ready for display.

To take on such a lengthy and labor-intensive process for one, let alone three, finished pieces highlighting a specific tissue in ways never before attempted would be a huge risk. It was also clear that such a feat could not be completed in time for the 2018 Fascia Research Congress, to be hosted in Berlin. It was decided to extend the project into a three-year plan and initially produce smaller, proof-of-concept pieces. And so the Fascial Net Plastination Project (FNPP) was born. In January of 2018 an international team of 14 bodyworkers and movement specialists, all with prior dissection skills, arrived in Guben for five days and got to work producing these pieces under the supervision of Robert Schleip, Carla Stecco, and Vladimir Chereminskiy, with assistance from John Sharkey. In July the team would return, enlarged by additional volunteers as word and support of the project began to grow (Figure 3.32).

One thing that was clear from the beginning was that this was going to be a deep learning process for everyone. Fascial dissection has its own way of working and so do the craftspeople and processes at the Plastinarium. Each would have to learn and adapt from each other, and

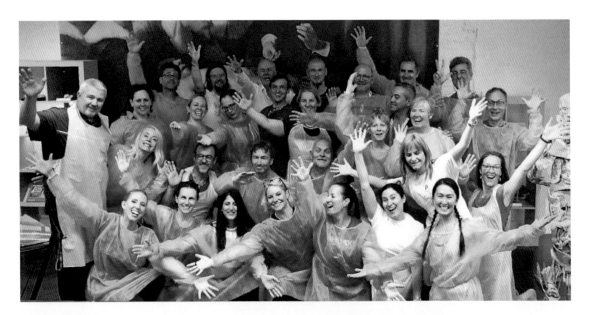

Figure 3.32
The FNPP Team at the end of the June Round of dissections. The pieces they created would become the centerpieces of the exhibition, Fascia in a NEW LIGHT. *Left to right, back row:* Bruce Schonfeld, Mika Pihlman, Robert Schleip, Tilo Heinrich, Bernd Michel, Andreas Haas, Johannes Freiberg. *Third row:* Stefan Westerback, Jihan Adem, Lauri Nemetz, Carla Stecco, Vladimir Chereminskiy, Tuulia Luomala, Anthony Chrisco, Tracey Mellor, Eric Franklin. *Second row:* Elizabeth Larkham, Walter Dorigo, Markus Friedlin, Gary Carter, Beverley Johnson, Cínta Báril, Birgit Frank. *First row:* Rachelle L. Clauson, Tjasa Cerovsek Landes, Einat Almog, Gina Tacconi-Moore, Alison Slater, Sivan Navot, Jo Phee.
Reproduced with permission from The Fascial Net Plastination Project, www.fasciaresearchsociety.org/plastination.

in some cases invent new approaches to bring these pieces to life (as it were). Not every new approach worked, but most of them did. The end result was ten distinct pieces that surpassed everyone's expectations. One piece includes our old friend from the beginning of this chapter, the iliotibial band (see Figures 3.2 and 3.3), and was produced by the combined efforts of Carla Stecco, Tjasa Cerovsek Landes, and Gary Carter.

Gary Carter began his professional life as an illustrator and graphic designer. He would eventually become director of a design and exhibition firm. There he often employed the scalpel of designers everywhere, the X-Acto knife, to build models and mock-ups of his designs. Eventually, he would leave this career path, open a gym, become a yoga teacher, structural integrator, myofascial anatomy teacher, and explorer of his own ideas in dissection labs for nearly two decades. This unique set of skills and experience would culminate in his volunteering for the FNPP and playing a key role in the development and design of the first fascia-focused whole-body plastinate. But first, there was that pesky IT band to deal with.

The goal was to show the reality of the IT band as part of the whole fascia lata, rather than as a separate, isolated structure as is typically

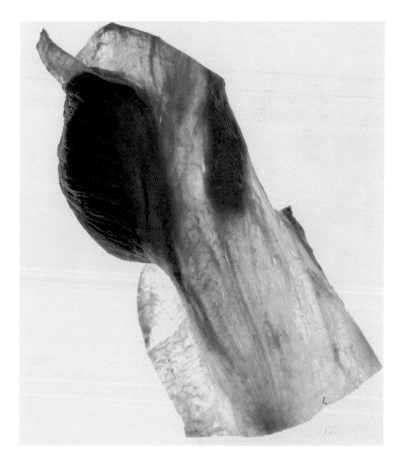

Figure 3.33
The plastinated fascia lata, with the tensor fascia lata and gluteus maximus intact and invested into the structure, including the visible thickening better known as the IT band. Note its relationship to the whole leg, rather than a discrete part.
Photo by Rachelle Clauson. Reproduced with permission from The Fascial Net Plastination Project, www.fasciaresearchsociety.org/plastination.

done. The plan was to separate all the muscle tissues of the thigh from the top of the iliac crest to just above the knee. The entry point for incision was along the sartorius. Then the muscle tissue was removed carefully, a few fibers at a time. Five days later the dissection was done, and the continuity of the IT band with the gluteus maximus and tensor fascia lata preserved. This was followed by the six-month bath and final positioning. The resulting plastinate (Figure 3.33) became one of the highlights, along with the pericardium (Figure 3.34) of Fascia in a NEW LIGHT, a special exhibition of the ten initial fascial plastinates.

Co-produced by Gary and FNPP dissection team member and media coordinator Rachelle Clauson, Fascia in a NEW LIGHT was a highlight of both the 2018 Berlin Fascia Research Congress and subsequent osteopathic conference (Figure 3.35). Visited by an estimated 2,000 people during its one-week showing, the exhibit has been digitally preserved for all to see. Lauri Nemetz, one of the FNPP dissectors, offered the use of Otocast, an app providing narrated audiovisual guides, and you can use it to view this exhibit right now. Use the QR code (Figure 3.36) to download the free Otocast app, type in the keyword "fascia" and access a complete tour of the exhibit in picture, print, and narration in three languages. And the next time you are in Berlin, you can visit BODY WORLDS and see some of these pieces that are now on permanent display.

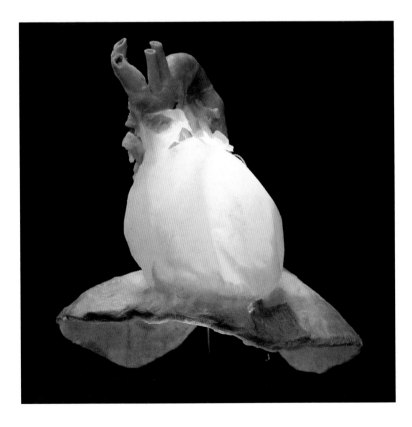

Figure 3.34
The pericardium sitting atop and with fibers continuous with the diaphragm.
Photo by Stefan Westerback. Reproduced with permission from The Fascial Net Plastination Project, www.fasciaresearchsociety.org/plastination.

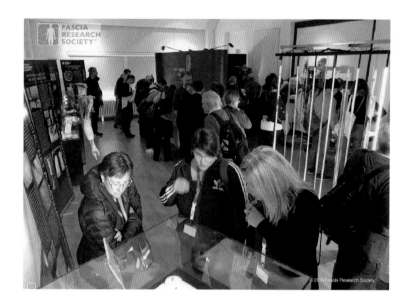

Figure 3.35
Fascia in a NEW LIGHT
exhibition, Berlin 2018.
Photo by author. Reproduced
with permission from The Fascial
Net Plastination Project, www.
fasciaresearchsociety.org/plastination.

This success ensured the next phase of the project.

Enter Freya

While talks had been ongoing, it was shortly after the 2018 Fascia Research Congress that Robert, Gary, and key players from BODY WORLDS and the Plastinarium met to discuss how to create the first whole-body fascial plastinate. If the goal was to show only the fascia, what would keep those empty fascial pockets open to display the empty space? How would it maintain its form and stability? Maybe one day those issues will also be overcome. For now, it was decided that the goal should be to create a "fascia-focused" whole-body plastinate rather than a "fascia-only" specimen as originally conceived. This limitation actually opened up new possibilities for showing the fascia in relationship to the other more recognized aspects of the body and in doing so truly highlighted its place as the tissue of connection.

Figure 3.36
QR Code for the Otocast app. Access the entire Fascia in a NEW LIGHT exhibition by downloading the app and searching "fascia." There are no fees.
Reproduced with permission from The Fascial Net Plastination Project, www.fasciaresearchsociety.org/plastination.

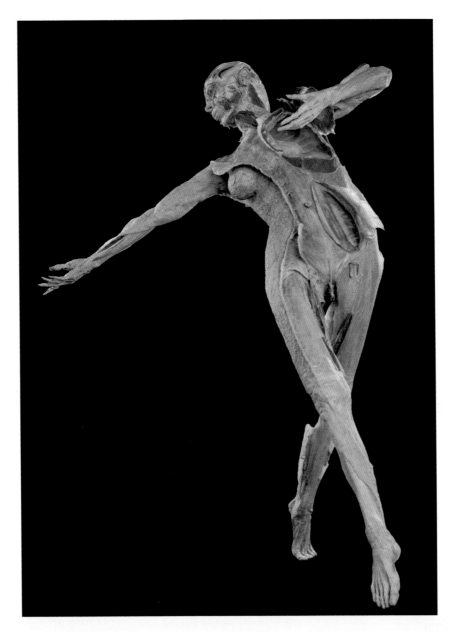

Figure 3.37
FR:EIA (Fascia Revealed: Educating Interconnected Anatomy) is the world's first 3-D human fascia plastinate. It was created at Dr. Gunther von Hagens' Plastinarium in Guben Germany, by his BODY WORLDS team in collaboration with the Fascia Research Society.
© www.BODYWORLDS.com/FR:EIA.

Vladimir Chereminskiy prepared the initial design based on classical anatomy concepts. After more discussion, it would fall to Gary and his design skills to fashion a more fluid design, and one that would include all ten prior pieces. In the following weeks and months, he would design and redesign the schematic for the final piece, incorporating ideas from consulted anatomy experts who included Dr. Chereminskiy, Gil Hedley, Tom Myers, Robert Schleip, John Sharkey, Carla Stecco, and Jaap van der Wal. It would also have to definitively display the one quality that every expert consulted insisted upon – "continuity." Achieving this would require dozens upon dozens of designs and redesigns of cardboard and paper mock-ups, and even real-life modeling on other team members. There could be no margin for error in the final dissection phase.

Then there was the body herself.

The female specimen was specially chosen by Angelina Whalley and quickly became an integral partner of the team. She was given the name "Freya," named after the Norse Goddess of Love and Beauty (and, strangely, also gold and war). Dissector Jihan Adem observed, "We are now a team of five."

Gary Carter elaborated:

All the way through the process, and all of us said this, that there is something about Freya that drove it and led it. We couldn't go any faster than she was going to allow. Her tissues would even hold us back in certain stages. If we went in there

with an agenda and said: "Right! We know what we're doing, we know the anatomy, we're going to go in and do this specific thing exactly this way," something in her would slow us down. We'd come across an issue, or something that would stop us and we'd have to regroup, think differently and slowly start again.

So very slowly, Freya began to take shape.

Positioned like a dancer, the result is exceptionally graceful. Showcasing the continuity of fascia from head to foot in long sweeping lines and spirals she evokes a sense of movement and showcases the dynamic elegance of the fascial system (Figure 3.37). Proclaimed Angelina Whalley – "It looks like BODY WORLDS has a new beauty."

So taken was Dr. Whalley with the final result that she rechristened her FR:EIA, an acronym for Fascia Revealed: Educating Interconnected Anatomy, and unveiled her to the world on 24 November 2021 in a special press conference and mini-symposium held at the BODY WORLDS museum in Berlin. The event was streamed worldwide (BODY WORLDS 2021), representing a crowning achievement for everyone involved, as well as the long line of anatomists through the centuries that led up to this moment. The study of fascial anatomy is here to stay, and permanently on display.

So far we have spent a lot a lot of brain power on the fascial anatomy of the musculoskeletal system. Does the fascia of the body connect into the brain? It turns out it does!

The myodural bridge – connecting the body to the brain

An actual soft-tissue connection between the posterior aspects of the atlas and axis and cervical dura mater was first published almost 100 years ago (Von Lanz 1929). A subsequent follow-up study (Kahn et al. 1992) found a connective-tissue bridge linking the dura mater to the rectus capitis posterior minor. Further examination revealed similar fibrous connections between the dura and the rectus capitis posterior major and obliquus capitis inferior (Figures 3.38 and 3.39).

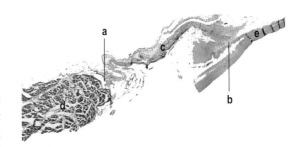

Figure 3.39

Hematoxylin and eosin stain; right side sagittal section of the connection between the rectus capitis posterior major (RCPma) muscle and the cervical dura mater in a female cadaveric specimen. Histological analysis depicts soft-tissue connection inserting into the belly of the RCPma (a) and the posterior aspect of the cervical dura mater (b). Also shown are the sensory receptors (c) which create the soft-tissue communication between the RCPma (d) and the posterior cervical dura mater (e).

Reprinted from Scali et al. (2013) with permission from Elsevier.

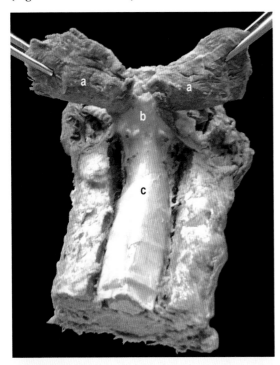

Figure 3.38

Image of a cervical spine laminectomy revealing the dural attachment of the rectus capitis posterior major muscles (a) and the cervical dura mater of the spinal cord (c) occurring via the fascia at b.

Reprinted from Scali et al. (2013) with permission from Elsevier.

Another histological study of this connection (Scali et al. 2013) also confirmed not only the existence of this structure but also the presence of proprioceptive nerve endings within the fibrous connecting tissues. More than mere fascial anchoring, the presence of these nerve endings clearly suggests that a real-time transmission of tensional forces in the head and neck to the dura is at work in this junction. It is further hypothesized that this relationship does not only regulate messages of dural tension but also the flow of cerebrospinal fluid.

The smooth functioning of this mechanical communication node between the myofascial body and nervous system has potential clinical implications and, for the purposes of this book, serves as a fitting segue to move from myofascial anatomy to a fascial exploration of the nervous system.

References

Benjamin M (2009) The fascia of the limbs and back—a review. J Anat. January; 214 (1) 1–18.

Benjamin M, Kaiser E and Milz S (2008) Structure-function relationships in tendons: A review. J Anat. March; 212 (3) 211–228.

BODY WORLDS (2021) Unveiling of FR:EIA. Fascia revealed: Educating Interconnected Anatomy. [Video] Available: www.youtube.com/watch?v=vCzX0c_D6kY [May 18, 2022].

Bogduk N (1980) The reappraisal of the human lumbar erector spinae. J Anat. October; 131 (Pt 3) 525–540.

Bogduk N, Wilson W S and Tynan W (1982) The human lumbar dorsal rami. J Anat. March; 134 (Pt 2) 383–397.

Borg T K and Caulfield J B (1980) Morphology of connective tissue in skeletal muscle. Tissue Cell. 12 (1) 197–207.

Detton A J (2016) Grant's Dissector, 16th edn. Philadelphia, PA: Wolters Kluwer.

Douglas J (1707) Myographiae Comparatae Specimen. London, UK: Printed by W B for G Strachan.

Findley T (2013) Recent advances in fascia research: Implications for sports medicine. Lecture at Connect 2013 Connective Tissues in Sports Medicine conference, University of Ulm, Germany, April 12–14, 2013. Published on DVD in the Collection "Fascia and Sports Medicine." Pittsburgh, PA: Singing Cowboy Productions.

Gray H (1893) Gray's Anatomy: Surgical and Descriptive, 13th edn. Lea Brothers, p. 39e1.

Huijing P A (2007) Epimuscular myofascial force transmission: A historical review and implications for new research. International Society of Biomechanics Muybridge Award Lecture, Taipei, 2007. J Biomech. January; 42 (1) 9–21.

Hukins D W, Aspden R M and Hickey D S (1990) Thoracolumbar fascia can increase efficiency of the erector spinae muscles. Clin Biomech. (Bristol, Avon). February; 5 (1) 30–34.

Kahn J L, Sick H and Kortiké J G (1992) Les espaces intervértébraux postérieurs de la jointure crânio-rachidienne. [The posterior intervertebral spaces of the craniovertebral joint]. Acta Anat (Basel). 144 (1) 65–70.

Langevin H M, Stevens-Tuttle D, Fox J R et al. (2009) Ultrasound evidence of altered lumbar connective tissue structure in human subjects with chronic low back pain. BMC Musculoskelet Disord. December; 10, 151.

Liem T, Tozzi P and Chila A (eds) (2017) Fascia in the Osteopathic Field. Edinburgh, UK: Handspring Publishing.

Luchau T (2016) Advanced Myofascial Techniques: Neck, Head, Spine and Ribs, Volume 2. Edinburgh, UK: Handspring Publishing.

Mense S (2019) Innervation of the thoracolumbar fascia. Eur J Transl Myol. September; 29 (3) 8297.

Myers T W (1997) The "anatomy trains." J Bodyw Mov Ther. January; 1 (2) 91–101.

Netter F H, MD (2014) Atlas of Human Anatomy, 6th edn. Philadelphia, PA: Saunders Elsevier.

Passerieux E, Rossignol R, Chopar A et al. (2006) Structural organization of the perimysium in bovine skeletal muscle: Junctional plates and associated intracellular subdomains. J Struct Biol. May; 154 (2) 206–216.

Purslow P P (2010) Muscle fascia and force transmission. J Bodyw Mov Ther. October; 14 (4) 411–417.

Scali F, Pontell M E, Enix D E and Marshall E (2013) Histological analysis of the rectus capitis posterior major's myodural bridge. Spine J. May; 13 (5) 558–563.

Schuenke M D, Vleeming A, Van Hoof T and Willard F H (2012) A description of the lumbar interfascial triangle and its relation with the lateral raphe: Anatomical constituents of load transfer through the lateral margin of the thoracolumbar fascia. J Anat. December; 221 (6) 568–576.

Stecco A, Gilliar W, Hill R et al. (2013) The anatomical and functional relation between gluteus maximus and fascia lata. J Bodyw Mov Ther. October; 17 (4) 512–517.

Stecco C (2015) Functional Atlas of the Human Fascial System. Edinburgh, UK: Churchill Livingstone Elsevier.

Stecco C, Stern R, Porzionato A et al. (2011) Hyaluronan within fascia in the etiology of myofascial pain. Surg Radiol Anat. December; 33 (10) 891–896.

Still A T (1899 [2015]) Philosophy of Osteopathy. Create Space Independent Publishing Platform.

van der Wal J (2009) The architecture of the connective tissue in the musculoskeletal system–an often overlooked functional parameter as to proprioception in the locomotor apparatus. Int J Ther Massage Bodywork. December; 2 (4) 9–23.

Vleeming A (2017) The functional coupling of the deep abdominal and paraspinal muscles Lecture at Connect 2017 Connective Tissues in Sports Medicine conference, University of Ulm, Germany, March 16–19.

Vleeming A, Pool-Goudzwaard A L, Stoeckart R et al. (1995) The posterior layer of the thoracolumbar fascia. Its function in load transfer from spine to legs. Spine (Phila Pa 1976). April; 20 (7) 753–758.

von Lanz T (1929) Uber die Ruchensmarkshaute. I. Die konstruktive Form der harten Haut des menschlichen Ruckenmarkes und ihrer Bander. [The structural form of the hard skin of the human spinal cord and its bands]. Arch Entwickl Mech Org. 118, 252–307.

Weisman M H, Haddad M, Lavi N and Vulfsons S (2014) Surface electromyographic recordings after passive and active motion along the posterior myofascial kinematic chain in healthy male subjects. J Bodyw Mov Ther. July; 18 (3) 452–461.

Wilke J, Krause F, Vogt L and Banzer W (2016) What is evidence-based about myofascial chains: A systematic review. Arch Phys Med Rehabil. March; 97 (3) 454–461.

Willard F H, Vleeming A, Schuenke M D, Danneels L and Schleip R (2012) The thoracolumbar fascia: Anatomy, function and clinical considerations. J Anat. December; 221 (6) 507–536.

Wilson L (1987) William Harvey's Prelections: The performance of the body in the Renaissance theater of anatomy. Representations (Berkeley). Winter; 17, 62–95.

Wilson W J E (1892) Wilson's Anatomist's Vade Mecum: A System of Human Anatomy, 11th edn, ed. Henry C. Clark. Churchill, p. 228.

Wood Jones F (1920) The principles of anatomy as seen in the hand. Philadelphia, PA: P. Blakiston's Son & Co., p. 160.

Zorn A and Hodeck K (2011) Walk with elastic fascia. In: Dalton E (ed.) Dynamic Body: Exploring Form, Expanding Function. Oklahoma, OK: Freedom from Pain Institute.

Further reading

Joffe S N (2014) Andreas Vesalius: The Making, The Madman, and the Myth. Bloomington, Indiana: AuthorHouse™ LLC.

Langevin H M and Huijing P A (2009) Communicating about fascia: History, pitfalls, and recommendations. Int J Ther Bodywork. December; 2 (4) 3–8.

Myers T W (2014) Anatomy Trains: Myofascial Meridians for Manual & Movement Therapists, 3rd edn. Edinburgh, UK: Churchill Livingstone Elsevier.

O'Keefe Aptowicz C (2015) Dr. Mütter's Marvels: A True Tale of Intrigue and Innovation at the Dawn of Modern Medicine. New York, NY: Avery.

Paoletti S (2006) The Fasciae: Anatomy, Dysfunction & Treatment. Seattle, Washington: Eastland Press.

Porter R (2003) Blood & Guts: A Short History of Medicine. London, UK: Norton.

Still A T (1897) Autobiography of Andrew T. Still. 2016 reprint edition. London, UK: Forgotten Books.

Tarshis J (1969) Andreas Vesalius: Father of Modern Anatomy. New York, NY: The Dial Press.

Tittel K (2015) Muscle Slings in Sport: Analysing Movements in Various Disciplines from a Functional-Anatomical Point of View. Munich, Germany: Kiener Press.

Wood Jones F (1943) Structure and Function as Seen in the Foot. London, UK: Baillière, Tindall & Cox.

4

The mind's first step to self-awareness must be through the body.

—Dr. George A. Sheehan

Introduction

This morning you woke up and maybe stretched a bit. Feeling a tug here or a pull there and moving your body just so before getting out of bed. You did not think about it, you just felt it and moved accordingly. You felt the solidity of the floor under the soles of your feet as you padded to the kitchen. You held your glass with just enough pressure so that you did not drop it into the sink or squeeze it so tightly that it cracked in your hand. You used just the right amount of torque to turn on the water faucet. And then you drank the glass of water. And you did that all without a single conscious thought.

You did not need to think about these things because you could feel yourself doing them. Ian Waterman cannot do any of these things without thinking about them because he cannot feel them. But Ian is not paralyzed. Ian Waterman has lost his proprioception.

The man who lost his body

In 1971, Ian was 19 years old and working in a butcher shop in England. One day at work he cut himself and shortly thereafter began to lose sensation in his body, so much so that he collapsed. Waking up in the hospital he could not even feel the bed beneath him. To Ian it was as if he was floating above the bed. To quote Ian:

"[There were] strange sensations in the collar area, the cuff and the ankle and ripping sensations across my stomach."

At first nobody, not even the doctors, knew what was happening to Ian. It is now believed that it was an undiagnosed fever that triggered an autoimmune response that destroyed all the sensory nerves below his neck. It was not the case that Ian could not move his body – his motor nerves were undamaged – but he could not control his movements. The innate sense of feeling his physical body was missing. His proprioception was gone.

In the original Latin, proprioception means "to grasp one's self." Famed neurologist Oliver Sacks defined it as "the unconscious sense that allows you to move normally." Also called kinesthesia, proprioception is so intrinsic to the experience of being in the physical world that most people do not even know that they have it. Underlying every movement and gesture, proprioception is the true sixth sense.

Here is a quick test of proprioception: Close your eyes and touch your nose. Unless you have been drinking adult beverages you probably aced it on the first try. Ian Waterman could not even do that much. There was no sensory information coming from Ian's peripheral nerves to complete the feedback loop with his brain.

With no hope for a neurological recovery, his doctors believed he would spend the rest of his life in a wheelchair.

Working through his despair, Ian was determined to find another way and to do whatever it took to have a normal life again. After spending several frustratingly unsuccessful weeks trying to work out how to do something as simple as sit up in bed, he had a sudden hunch that if he could visualize the movement with his mind that he could, with his will power and concentration, replicate it with his body.

He practiced seeing a sequence of movements in his mind. In this case, the movements were flexing his head, bringing his shoulders forward, flexing his torso, and so on. Sometimes the appropriate muscle would even twitch while he was visualizing. Soon Ian was able to sit up for the first time. He was so excited by his accomplishment that he immediately fell back down onto the bed. But this brief moment of victory gave Ian all the resolve he needed to continue. He knew that if he could plan the movement and structure the sequence clearly in his mind, he could then replicate it with his body. The other key, beyond his thinking, was his sight. Ian had to be able to see what he was doing in order to will his body to follow along.

While his gait has been described as lumbering – Ian refers to his style of walking as "controlled falling" – he has mastered the use of his upper body. His mastery includes the use of hand gestures when conversing. By and large, he appears normal. Of the ten known cases of loss of proprioception, Ian is the only person who has managed to achieve such finesse. It is speculated that perhaps this was due to his young age (all the other cases affected much older individuals).

Whatever the reason, Ian has moved on to have a full life again. However, he still has to plan his every move and observe his body in order to accomplish it. To this day Ian sleeps with a light on because if he were to wake up in darkness he would not be able to get out of bed.

The nerves responsible for proprioception are sensory nerves and they are embedded in the fascia.

Anatomy of a nerve

Like a fiber optic cable, the nerve is an enclosed bundle of axons that provides a structured pathway for the transmission of nerve impulses from the brain via the central nervous system to the peripheral nervous system, and vice versa, in an efferent–afferent feedback loop of motion and sensation. The axons are projections of the neurons themselves, transmitting electrical signals from the brain. It should be noted that the faster, myelinated axons are also referred to as nerve fibers (Figure 4.1). All axons, myelinated or unmyelinated, terminate in different places in the body, such as muscles, organs, glands, etc., and in the case of sensory nerves they terminate in the fascia.

Like muscles, nerves are encased in fascia, and in the same configuration (Bove 2008). This fascia is often referred to specifically as the meningeal fascia. While it may be useful to distinguish it this way it is still contiguous with the whole of the fascial system. The basic anatomy of all peripheral nerves is a three-layer fascial arrangement of tubes and bundles of tubes (Figure 4.2), just like the muscles. Each axon is wrapped in a layer of loose connective tissue called the endoneurium. The endoneurium runs the entire length of the axon. To give that some perspective, the longest axons in the

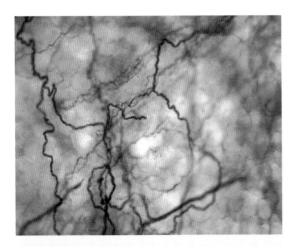

Figure 4.1
A dense network of nerve fibers in the thoracolumbar fascia of a rat. The surface area of the picture represents 0.5 mm (less than a tenth of an inch).
Reproduced from Tesarz et al. 2011 with permission from Elsevier.

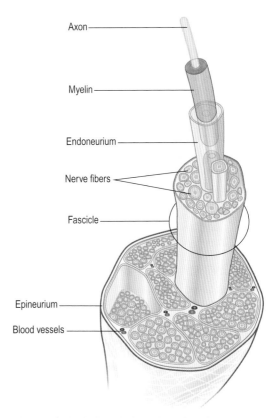

Figure 4.2
Cross-section of a typical spinal nerve. Note the similarities to the structure of the muscle (see Figure 3.11).

body belong to the sciatic nerve, which forms at the sacral plexus (L4–S3) and runs all the way to the end of the big toe. That is one long tube. Endoneurium also contains the fluid of the nerve, considered analogous to the cerebrospinal fluid of the central nervous system.

Groups of axons are then bundled together into fascicles by the perineurium. The perineurium is a dense layer of connective tissue that can be anywhere between one to six layers thick. These fascicles are then wrapped in another sheath called the epineurium that encloses the entire nerve.

While all of the enveloping connective layers are a mixture of collagen fibers and glycocalyx (a polysaccharide that plays both an adhesive and an immune role for the nerve), the epineurium is a looser areolar layer that allows the nerve a healthy degree of stretch and slide within

its environment. The layers also help to cushion the nerve during compression. Anatomically the epineurium is continuous with the dura mater (see Chapter 5), making another fascial connection to the brain.

While the physical parallels of nerve structure to muscle structure should be obvious, what is far less obvious is that in a typical muscle nerve there are three times as many sensory neurons as there are motor neurons (Figure 4.3), each with their own axons, of course. This ratio seems to indicate that the

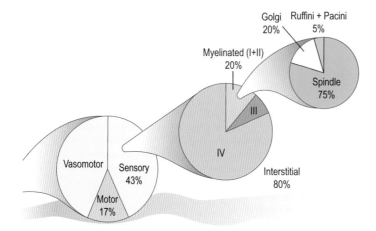

Figure 4.3
In the typical muscle nerve there are three times as many sensory nerves as there are motor nerves. Of those, around 80 per cent of the sensory information comes from interstitial nerves.

body's need for sensory awareness and refinement is greater than its need for motor control. Why else devote so much bandwidth to it?

These sensory nerves, or sensory receptors, are also called fascial mechanoreceptors – "fascial" because they are so abundant within the fascial system and "mechanoreceptors" because they are stimulated by the mechanical sensation of pressure and vibration. Taken collectively, the sheer amount of sensory information being relayed through this network is potentially greater than even that of the skin or the power of sight. This led researcher Robert Schleip (2011), and since then many others, to refer to fascia as the body's largest sensory organ. How large? Somewhere in the neighborhood of over 250 million nerve endings.

For those of you who want to do the math, it's not like we could count them all individually; this number was first estimated at 100 million (Grunwald 2017) based on numbers from the data set of Tanaka and Kawamura (1992), which lists the total mass of dense collagenous tissue of an average male as 5 kilograms. However, when the mass of the loose connective tissue is added

(to include the larger fascial system and using the same data set) that increases the overall fascial mass to 12.5 kilograms or 2½ times larger. This number is still, of course, an estimate. It is also based on the notion that the superficial fascia is as equally innervated as the deep fascia. Given that there are several studies that showing superficial fascia to be *more* highly innervated (Tesarz et al. 2011, Benetazzo et al. 2011), the actual number may turn out to be higher still.

Fascial mechanoreceptors

There are five types of fascial mechanoreceptors for the relay of all this proprioceptive sensory information.

Muscle spindles

Muscle spindles (Figure 4.4) are sensory receptors located in the belly of the muscle. They are encapsulated in a layer of fascia that is actually an extension of the perimysium itself (Stecco C. 2015). Arranged in parallel with the power-producing, extrafusal muscle fibers, muscle spindles are both stretch and speed receptors with primary and secondary endings. The primary

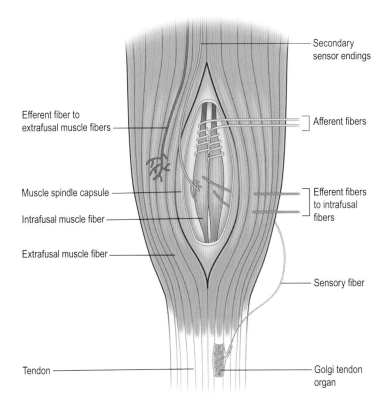

Secondary sensor endings

Efferent fiber to extrafusal muscle fibers

Afferent fibers

Muscle spindle capsule

Efferent fibers to intrafusal fibers

Intrafusal muscle fiber

Extrafusal muscle fiber

Sensory fiber

Tendon

Golgi tendon organ

Figure 4.4
The muscle spindle, embedded in the perimysium and interacting with the collagen network.

endings are myelinated and responsible for quickly relaying data about both the speed and size of changes in overall muscle length. Secondary endings can sense only changes in length, not velocity.

Under a prolonged stretch, such as carrying a suitcase or a heavy bag over a distance, the muscle spindles of the muscles under load will activate in order to actually increase the strength of muscle contraction to compensate for muscle fatigue.

Golgi receptors

Golgi receptors (Figure 4.5) are found throughout the deep fascia. However, just to make things confusing, when located around myotendinous junctions, they are referred to as Golgi tendon

organs. When found in ligaments, they are referred to as Golgi end organs. According to van der Wal (2009), however, there is no inherent difference between a muscle, a tendon, or a ligament receptor.

It should also be noted that only 10 per cent of Golgi receptors are actually found within the tendon. The other 90 per cent are found in the aforementioned ligaments, joint capsules, aponeurotic attachment sites, and the muscular portion of the myotendinous junctions.

Golgi receptors monitor tension level in ligaments and tendons. When stimulated by slow stretching, Golgi receptors respond by slowing the firing rate of specific alpha motor neurons,

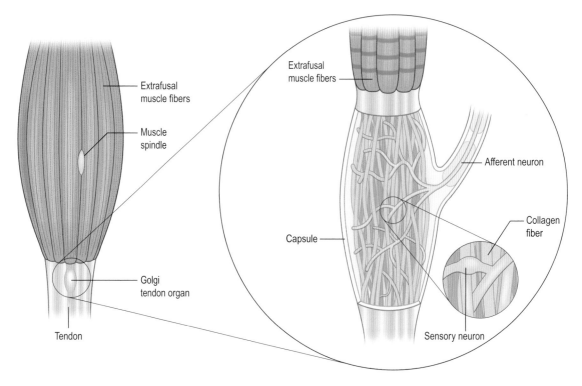

Figure 4.5
The Golgi tendon receptor where the muscle meets the bone.

generating a decrease in the tonus of the muscle. This is believed to be a protective measure, to keep from overdoing it, but this only happens when there is active muscle contraction. That is because Golgi receptors are arranged in series with muscle fibers and tendons, and tendons are much stiffer. Because of this arrangement, passive stretching tends to affect only the muscle, the relatively relaxed fibers of which will "soak up" most of the stretch. However, small, isometric contractions are sufficient to engage the Golgi receptors and this contract–relax mechanism is what underlies the efficacy of proprioceptive

neuromuscular facilitation (PNF) and other similar therapies.

Finally, there are the rarer Golgi–Mazzoni corpuscles, which monitor compression forces in joints. While abundant in the knee, they have also been discovered in the retinacula of the ankle (Stecco C. et al. 2010).

Pacini receptors

Also known as lamellar corpuscles, the egg-shaped Pacini receptors (Figure 4.6) are found in the more tendinous portions of the myotendinous

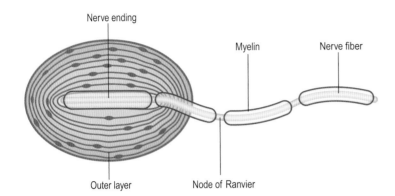

Nerve ending

Myelin

Nerve fiber

Outer layer

Node of Ranvier

Figure 4.6
A Pacini receptor or corpuscle. There are an estimated 3,000 Pacini corpuscles in each fingertip alone.

junctions, deep capsular layer of the joints, the epimysium, spinal ligaments, and facet joints. Much smaller receptors called paciniform corpuscles are located in the interosseus membranes.

Pacini receptors respond to sudden, rapid changes in pressure and vibration by increasing both proprioception and motor control. Given their high density in the spine, it is likely that stimulation of the Pacini receptors accounts for some of the beneficial effect after a high-velocity, low-amplitude (HVLA) chiropractic-style adjustment.

Curiously, lamellar corpuscles have also been found in some of the abdominal viscera, notably the pancreas (Handwiki 2022). It is thought that the ability of Pacini receptors to detect vibrations (especially low-frequency sounds and heavy air movement) is responsible for that distinctive feeling in the gut when in the presence of a heavy bass sound at a rock or symphony orchestra concert.

Ruffini receptors

Ruffini receptors (Figure 4.7) are found in the ligaments of peripheral joints, the dura mater, the fibrous outer layer of joint capsules and tissues

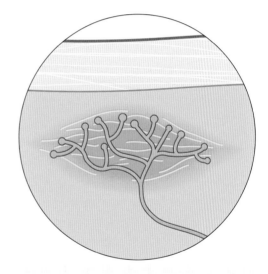

Figure 4.7
A Ruffini receptor.

associated with regular stretching, the skin, and superficial fascia. They monitor vibration, pressure, and especially shearing forces.

Ruffini receptors also respond to sustained changes in pressure with shear. This is often referred to in manual therapy as melting pressure. When properly stimulated, they create a global decrease in muscle tonus. Basically, when Ruffini receptors fire, you chill out. They are also very sensitive to both shearing forces and lateral stretch.

Interstitial receptors

Interstitial receptors (Figure 4.8) are the most abundant and mysterious mechanoreceptors in the fascia. Interstitial receptors are also called free nerve endings and account for almost 80 per cent of all sensory nerve fibers in a typical motor nerve. There are both myelinated Type III fibers and the unmyelinated Type IV fibers, also known as C fibers. Free nerve endings are found nearly everywhere throughout the body. They surround hair follicles and are also inside bone, and everywhere in between. They are abundant in the shearing, sliding zones between the superficial and the deep fascia.

Interstitial receptors give the body constant feedback about mechanical changes of tension, stress, sensations, temperature, and more. Some interstitial receptors perform autonomic functions and help to regulate heart rate and blood pressure. They also assist the nervous system in fine-tuning the regulation of blood flow (Figure 4.8).

Responding to extremely light pressure (like a hair follicle) and also very heavy pressure (think periosteum), stimulated free nerve endings can increase proprioceptive sensitivity. They also function as thermoreceptors, with the most common type of free nerve endings being the nociceptors. Nociceptive free nerve endings are often polymodal, responding not just to mechanical stimuli but also to all sorts of stimuli such as heat or cold and chemicals associated with tissue damage and disease. It has also been suggested that hyperactivated free nerve endings are a source of chronic myofascial pain (Stecco A. et al. 2013).

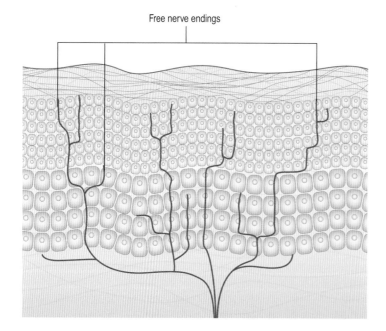

Free nerve endings

Figure 4.8

Interstitial or free nerve endings, which are responsible for 80 per cent of our sensory input.

This suggestion is further reinforced by Mense (2019), who examined specimens of thoracolumbar fascia (TLF). In the several hundred specimens examined – mostly from rats but with some human samples as well, and despite employing numerous staining techniques – none of the corpuscular proprioceptors (spindles, Golgis, Ruffinis) were found. They found only Type IV free nerve endings. Quite the surprise given the TLF's presumed role of proprioception in the low back. One possible reason for this was that the region examined was restricted to 5 mm lateral to the spinous processes. It should also be noted that free nerve endings in rats and humans appear identical.

One other interesting insight from this data was the distribution of the free nerve endings, which was not uniform between the three layers of the TLF, with most nerve endings appearing in both the inner and outer layers.

Remember, when you step on the brake your life is in your foot's hands. (George Carlin)

An anatomical examination of 27 legs found an abundance of Pacini, Ruffini, and free nerve endings in the retinacula of the ankle (Stecco C. et al. 2010). These examinations also revealed the retinacula to have a complex, three-layered architecture, with connections to both muscle and bone and also a reinforcement of the deepest fascial layers. This seems inordinately complex for what has been regarded in classical anatomy as a passive stabilizer and pulley structure for tendons. While the connective tissue aspect does give retinacula a stabilizing role, their intricate structure and rich innervation suggest that they should be thought of as a proprioceptive organ as well, sensing the loading and movement of the foot and ankle joint and transmitting that kinesthetic and sensory information to the knee, hip, torso, and brain. Furthermore, "The retinaculum of the ankle is a dynamic structure, and stress (loading) makes it stronger and thicker" (Stecco C. 2020).

What About Piezo2?

In 2021 neuroscientist Armen Patapoutian PhD received the Nobel Prize in Physiology for his work in the discovery of a pressure-sensitive ion channel known as Piezo2. Piezo2 is essential to how cells respond to touch and the principal mechanotransduction channel for proprioception. More than just an ion channel, Piezo2 is a specialized protein molecule embedded in the cell membrane that allows some cells to respond to pressure and touch. Piezo2 is expressed in the proprioceptors innervating both muscle spindles and Golgi tendon organs. The lack of Piezo2 has been shown to create extremely uncoordinated movements in mice (Woo et al. 2015) and adults with scoliosis express a definite deficiency in the Piezo2 gene (Wu et al. 2020).

While the Nobel Prize is new (along with the work of Professor Patapoutian's prize-sharing colleague Dr David Julius on the temperature receptor/protein Piezo1), the research around Piezo2 is not, with Professor Patapoutian having first identified it in 2009. He also points out:

I want to emphasize there is a whole field of people working in this area. Specifically in my lab, there's a big group of young, enthusiastic, smart scientists, graduate students and post docs who actually do the work. I share this with all of them, of course. (Scripps Research Press Release 2021)

May his generosity and largesse toward his colleagues and coworkers be an example to us all.

Proprioception and pain

When it comes to pain, I have always said that "perception is nine-tenths of the law." What we perceive, and what we have the capacity to perceive, has an impact on our reality. When it comes to pain, this is sometimes quite literally true.

A study by Taimela et al. (1999) found that proprioception was impaired when lumbar fatigue was induced in both groups of healthy people and groups with low back pain (LBP). That should come as no surprise. What was surprising was that all patients with LBP displayed poorer proprioception than their healthy counterparts.

A comparison study of proprioception (Lee et al. 2010) between patients with LBP and healthy controls (people with no LBP) found a significant decrease in proprioception among the group with LBP, especially in rotational movements.

Both of those studies were on humans. A study on rats (Lambertz et al. 2008) used TTX (tetrodotoxin), a mild neurotoxin, to temporarily inhibit the myelinated nerves in the lumbar fascia. This left the nociceptive potential of free nerve endings unaltered. Rats that had their proprioception thus inhibited displayed strong pain reactions from the lightest stimulation on the affected areas.

Fascia, rather than muscle, was also shown to be the main source of pain in delayed onset muscle soreness (Gibson et al. 2009). By simulating downhill walking, human participants were subjected to repetitive, eccentric contraction strain in the lower leg. The following day a slightly hypertonic saline solution was used to produce a pain response. When the belly of the muscle in the affected area was injected, there was no pain response. When ultrasound imaging was used to accurately inject the solution into the fascial epimysium of the muscle, the pain response was positive.

Hypertonic saline solution, which produces a mild irritation, was also used in a study on the thoracolumbar fascia of humans (Schilder et al. 2014). It was discovered that the thoracolumbar fascia was more sensitive to pain sensations than the underlying erector spinae. These fascial sensations were most often described as burning, throbbing, and stinging. Overall, the conclusion was that fascia is the most pain-sensitive tissue in the low back, which certainly jibes with the Mense study as highlighted above.

Since these studies demonstrate a direct correlation between diminished proprioception and increased pain, it would seem a logical corollary that when proprioception is increased, pain is likewise diminished, or perhaps not. A 2014 systematic literature review by McCaskey et al. concluded that the evidence suggests no consistent benefit to adding proprioceptive training to improve function. However, in the same review he admitted: "There are few relevant good quality studies on proprioceptive exercises."

We need those good quality studies. Anecdotally I see in my clinical practice that careful, sensitive induction of proprioception combined with manual stimulation decreases pain levels and improves mobility.

I also know the value of heightened proprioception from my long-time yoga practice, although any system of movement with concentration such as t'ai chi, the Alexander Technique, the Feldenkrais Method®, and a variety of martial arts should engender this same awareness.

Far from being just a placebo effect – and there is nothing wrong with a good placebo effect – this instinctive knowing that involves the stimulation of the interstitial receptors goes far deeper into the body, into the even murkier waters of internal awareness, otherwise known as interoception.

Interoception – the seventh sense

Interstitial receptors are multimodal. That means they are capable of producing a wide variety of internal sensations. Not just pain, but sensations of hot, cold, hunger, thirst, itch, sensual touch, and so on. Collectively this is known as interoception. Interoception is defined as the awareness of one's own internal body state, our sense of the body's own internal signals. While it is just beginning to be understood, interoception is essential to our sense of embodiment, motivation, and well-being (Farb et al. 2015).

These sensations, triggered by the unmyelinated free nerve endings, are processed through the brain's insular cortex (Berlucchi & Aglioti 2010). Faulty interoceptive input is now thought to be involved across a wide spectrum of psychosomatic and somatoemotional disorders. Both anxiety and depression are accompanied by significant alterations in interoception (Paulus & Stein 2010), as are eating disorders like bulimia and anorexia.

A study of 214 college-age females (Peat & Muehlenkamp 2011) found that those who scored lower on measures of interoceptive ability also had higher levels of body dissatisfaction and were more likely to display symptoms of eating disorders.

It is further speculated that faulty interoception could also be at work in conditions like irritable bowel, fibromyalgia, and chronic fatigue syndromes.

Testing interoception

A simple and reliable test for interoceptive ability was developed by neuroscientist Hugh Critchley, and all it entails is becoming aware of your own heartbeat. Critchley et al. (2004) found that subjects who could most accurately guess the rate of their heartbeat also scored higher on other tests of interoceptive awareness.

You can do the test right now. All you need is a stopwatch. Your phone probably has one built in, or you can use a kitchen timer. Here are the steps:

1. Set the timer for one minute.

2. Sit in a comfortable position and take a few deep breaths.

3. Start the timer and count the number of heartbeats you feel. Write down that number.

4. Now repeat this same process while taking the pulse in either your wrist or neck. Wait two minutes and take your pulse again, and then average the two results.

5. Take the difference between the two counts. If, for example, the estimate was 60 and the pulse average was 80, the difference would be 20.

6. Divide that number 20, by the average pulse number 80. In this example the answer would be 0.25.

7. Subtract that number from 1. In this example the answer would be 0.75. The scores can be interpreted as follows:

- 0.80 or higher = very good interoception

- 0.600–0.79 = moderate interoception

- 0.59 or lower = poor interoception.

Improving interoception requires focused attention...

Physical activities that require more focused attention, as opposed to using the treadmill while watching videos, have the capacity to increase interoception. For example, daily yoga has been shown to bring about positive benefits in adolescents with eating disorders (Carei et al. 2010). Likewise, having to pay attention to one's physical therapy also seems to reap great dividends. This was ingeniously demonstrated by pain pioneer Lorimer Moseley (Moseley et al. 2008). In this trial patients receiving identical therapy for complex regional pain syndrome in the hand were divided into two groups. While neither group was allowed to observe the area being treated, the control group was allowed to read, listen to music, or be otherwise distracted during treatment.

The other group had to look at a photograph of a hand. The photograph was marked with numbers that were correlated with the stimulation sites. Patients had to give feedback based on where they felt the treatment – by the numbers, as it were. In every patient studied the results were the same. They showed that tactile discrimination along with tactile stimulation achieved a decrease in pain to a degree that tactile stimulation alone could not produce.

...for the therapist as well as the patient

But what about the focus of the tactile stimulationist, i.e., the therapist? Can their tactile focus make a difference on the recipient of touch? Certainly, our individual experiences of the many kinds of touch seem to indicate that we have the ability to perceive the cognitive-emotional state of the person who is touching us. While those experiences are usually multifactorial and context-dependant, a recent fMRI study (Cerritelli et al. 2017) indicates that indeed, this is exactly what we do.

The operators, the ones applying the touch, were put through a process designed to help them accurately reproduce just the right amount of touch to stimulate the afferent tactile C-fibers (hello interstitial receptors!). The exact amount of force was estimated, based on prior touch studies, to be 0.2 Newtons. The operators used a cylindrical device wired with force transducers tied to a visual feedback aide to practice delivering just the right amount of touch.

Since the subjects would be in an fMRI chamber, it was decided that the area of focus would be the malleolus, the bony prominences on either side of the ankle.

For the experimental phase, one group of operators was told to focus their attention on the feel of the tissue under their hands and prompted to give awareness to consistency, density, temperature, responsiveness, and motility. While motility usually refers to independent movement via metabolic energy, like your stomach, it is of interest to note that this paper defined motility as "myofascial movement."

The other group of operators was to focus on a series of beeps delivered at random intervals via headphones. Their focus would be on counting the number of beeps in each sequence, all while maintaining contact with the malleolus of the subject. There was a total of 40 subjects and each fMRI with touch was repeated five times. There were no reported imbalances in the quality of touch by the subjects in the fMRI, who overall rated the touch as "pleasant," and other similar qualities. What happened in the brain, however, was revelatory.

Nine regions of the brain were studied. The most active in both groups were the posterior cingulate cortex, the right inferior frontal gyrus, and the right insula (the insula being part of the interoceptive, salience network). While it was demonstrated that the insular cortex was active in all subjects there was a marked difference in the functional connectivity between the two groups. Those who received prolonged static touch from the operators focused on tactile awareness exhibiting greater connectivity. In other words, and to quote the authors of the paper:

...results showed that, if a particular cognitive status of the operator is sustained over time, it is able to elicit significant effects in the subjects' functional connectivity between areas processing the interoceptive and attentional value of touch. (Cerritelli et al. 2017)

So, for all you therapists out there reading this right now, what's going on in your head can make a big difference for your client or patient. Even if you never utter a single word.

And since this is a book about fascia, it is important to note this, from the "Further Considerations" part of the same paper:

...speculating on a plausible mechanism of action, we would argue that a touch focused on the myofascial movement would more accurately trigger the subject's CT afferent fibres receptors (i.e. low-threshold mechanoreceptors), starting a cascade of bottom-up neurobiological events ending with distinct involvement of specific areas and networks of the brain. In addition, modifying the afferent input through this type of touch would change the metabolic condition and thus it's interoceptive inflow, possibly producing a central effect in terms of functional connectivity. (Cerritelli et al. 2017)

Touch aside, all these studies indicate that what we pay attention to, and the quality of that attention, matters. That to which we bring our focused attention can amplify the desired result.

In mind–body medicine terms, this would be called mindfulness – and that involves our next port of call, the brain.

References

Benetazzo L, Bizzego A, DeCaro R et al. (2011) 3D reconstruction of the crural and thoracolumbar fasciae. Surg Radiol Anat. December; 33 (10) 855–862.

Berlucchi G and Aglioti S M (2010) The body in the brain revisited. Exp Brain Res. January; 200 (1) 25–35.

Bove G (2008) Epi-perineurial anatomy, innervation, and axonal nociceptive mechanisms. J Bodyw Mov Ther. July; 12 (3) 185–190.

Carei T R, Fyfe-Johnson A L, Breuner C C and Brown M A (2010) Randomized controlled clinical trial of yoga in the treatment of eating disorders. J Adolesc Health. April; 46 (4) 346–351.

Cerritelli F, Chiacchiaretta P, Gambi F and Ferretti A (2017) Effect of continuous touch on brain functional connectivity is modified by the operator's tactile attention. Front Hum Neurosci. July; 11, 368.

Critchley H D, Wiens S, Rotshtein P et al. (2004) Neural systems supporting interoceptive awareness. Nature Neurosci. February; 7 (2) 189–195.

Farb N, Daubenmier J, Price C J et al. (2015) Interoception, contemplative practice, and health. Front Psychol. June; 6, 763.

Gibson W, Arendt-Neilsen L, Taguchi T et al. (2009) Increased pain from muscle fascia following eccentric exercise: Animal and human findings. Exp Brain Res. April; 194 (2) 299–308.

Grunwald M (2017) Homo Hapticus. Munich: Droemer Verlag, p. 54.

Handwiki (2022) Biology: Lamellar corpuscle. Available: https://handwiki.org/wiki/ Biology:Lamellar_corpuscle [May 23, 2022].

Lambertz D, Hoheiseil U and Mense S (2008) Influence of a chronic myositis on rat spinal field potentials evoked by TTX-resistant unmyelinated skin and muscle afferents. Eur J Pain. August; 12 (6) 686–695.

Lee A S, Cholewicki J, Reeves N P et al. (2010) Comparison of trunk proprioception between patients with low back pain and healthy controls. Arch Phys Med Rehabil. September; 91 (9) 1327–1331.

McCaskey M A, Schuster-Amft C, Wirth B et al. (2014) Effects of proprioceptive exercises on pain and function in chronic neck- and low-back pain rehabilitation: A systematic literature review. BMC Musculoskelet Disord. November; 15, 382.

Moseley G L, Zalucki N M and Wiech K (2008) Tactile discrimination, but not tactile stimulation alone, reduces chronic limb pain. Pain. July; 137 (3) 600–608.

Mense S (2019) Innervation of the thoracolumbar fascia. Eur J Transl Myol. August; 29 (3) 8297.

Paulus M P and Stein M B (2010) Interoception in anxiety and depression. Brain Struct Funct. June; 214 (5–6), 451–463.

Peat C M and Muehlenkamp J J (2011) Self-objectification, disordered eating, and depression: A test of mediational pathways. Psychology of Women Quarterly. May; 35 (3) 441–450.

Schilder A, Hoheisel U, Magerl W et al. (2014) Sensory findings after stimulation of the thoracolumbar fascia with hypertonic saline suggest its contribution to low back pain. Pain. September; 155 (2) 222–231.

Schleip R (2011) Fascia as a sensory organ. In: Dalton E (ed.) Dynamic Body: Exploring Form Expanding Function. Freedom from Pain Institute, pp. 136–163.

Scripps Research Press Release (2021) Scripps Research neuroscientist Ardem Patapoutian receives 2021 Nobel Prize in Physiology. Available: www.scripps.edu/news-and-events/press-room/2021/20211004-ardem-patapoutian-wins-nobel-prize-in-medicine.html [April 29, 2022].

Stecco A, Gilliar W, Hill R et al. (2013) The anatomical and functional relation between gluteus maximus and the fascia lata. J Bodyw Mov Ther. October; 17 (4) 512–517.

Stecco C (2015) The Functional Atlas of the Human Fascial System. Edinburgh, UK: Churchill Livingstone Elsevier, p. 64.

Stecco C (2020) Fascial anatomy. In: Lesondak D and Akey A (eds) Fascia, Function, and Medical Applications. Boca Raton, FL: CRC Press/Taylor & Francis, p. 25.

Stecco C, Macchi V, Porzionato A et al. (2010) The ankle retinacula: Morphological evidence of the proprioceptive role of the fascial system. Cells Tissues Organs. 2010; February; 192 (3) 200–210.

Taimela S, Kankaanpää M M and Luoto S (1999) The effect of lumbar fatigue on the ability to sense a change in lumbar position. A controlled study. Spine. July; 24 (13) 1322–1327.

Tanaka G and Kawamura H (1992) Reference man models based on normal data from human populations. International Commission on Radiological Protection. Available: www.irpa.net/ irpa10/cdrom/00602.pdf [April 29, 2022].

Tesarz J, Hoheisel U, Wiedenhöfer B and Mense S (2011) Sensory innervation of the thoracolumbar fascia in rats and humans. Neuroscience. October; 194, 302–308.

van der Wal J (2009) The architecture of the connective tissue in the musculoskeletal system—an often overlooked functional parameter as to proprioception in the locomotor apparatus. J Bodyw Mov Ther. December; 2 (4) 9–23.

Woo S-H, Lukacs V, de Nooij J C et al. (2015) Piezo2 is the principal mechanotransduction channel for proprioception. Nat Neurosci. December; 18 (12) 1756–1762.

Wu Z, Wang Y, Xia C et al. (2020) Piezo2: A novel molecule involved in the development of AIS. Spine (Phila Pa 1976). February; 45 (3) E120–E125.

Further reading

Aranyosi I (2013) The Peripheral Mind: Philosophy of Mind and the Peripheral Nervous System. New York, NY: Oxford University Press.

BBC Horizon (1998) [documentary series] The man who lost his body.

Blakeslee S and Blakeslee M (2008) The Body Has a Mind of Its Own. New York, NY: Random House.

Cohen H (ed.) (1999) Neuroscience for Rehabilitation, 2nd edn. Philadelphia, PA: Lippincott Williams & Wilkins.

Cole J and Waterman I (1995) Pride and a Daily Marathon. Cambridge, MA: The MIT Press.

Craig A D (2002) How do you feel? Interoception: The sense of the physiological condition of the body. Nat Rev Neurosci. August; 3 (8) 655–666.

Mountcastle V C (2005) The Sensory Hand: Neural Mechanisms of Somatic Sensation. Cambridge, MA: Harvard University Press.

Purves D, Augustine G J, Fitzpatrick D et al. (eds) (2012) Neuroscience, 5th edn. Sunderland, MA: Sinauer Associates.

Radiolab [n.d.] [radio series] The butcher's assistant. WNYC Studios. Available: www.radiolab.org/story/91526-the-butchers-assistant [May 18, 2022].

Schleip R (2003) Fascial plasticity – a new neurobiological explanation. J Bodyw Mov Ther. January; 7 (1) 11–19 and April; 7 (2) 104–116.

Schleip R (2015) Fascia as a sensory organ. In: Schleip R (ed.) Fascia in Sport and Movement. Edinburgh, UK: Handspring Press, pp. 31.

5

Fascia and the Brain

When you deal with the fasciae you are doing business with the branch offices of the brain...

—Andrew Taylor Still

Introduction

One of the big focuses in the world of integrative medicine is mind–body medicine. How can we use the power of our thoughts and emotions to have a positive impact on our physical health and well-being? While that is a worthy question it does seem to me there is a top-down bias at work here that assumes the intelligence of the mind has primacy and agency over the intelligence of the body. If that were true, we might not have survived long enough to have created Western medicine.

I happily admit to having the other bias – body–mind medicine, if you will. It is impossible to be a clinician and not recognize how positive changes in the body involving pain levels, changes in movement patterns, and physical performance issues can positively influence mood and behavior.

There is a school of philosophy known as embodied cognition. Embodied cognition is the philosophical belief that human thinking is shaped by aspects of the body beyond the perception or independence of the brain. To simplify it even more, because we think with our brain which is a physical part of our body every thought we have is physical. There can be no other way. Without the body there is nothing to perceive and without the mind there is

no perceiver. Or, as Stephen A. Wainwright, Professor Emeritus of Biology at Duke University, put it: "Structure without function is a corpse. Function without structure is a ghost."

It is equally important to realize that the brain processes both in parallel and in series (Sigman & Dehaene 2008). There is so much going on in the brain at any one given moment – sensory input, autonomic monitoring, interoceptive awareness, motor control, organized and stray thoughts, and so on – one could not be consciously aware of all of it at any given moment, let alone process it. Awareness is different than reason. Reason tends to function linearly as a sequence of structured thoughts; therefore, we reason that the brain must work this way too, linearly, but perhaps it does not.

In reality, what we actually have is another partnership model between the mind and the body. It is a "both/and" system as opposed to an "either/or" system. While it is necessary and useful to study the systems of the body separately, I would argue that the split between the mind and the body is quite arbitrary and the division largely artificial.

René Descartes (1596–1650) is usually credited as the villain who created this division, but in truth he was a philosophical free spirit trying to live his life in reaction to his time.

During his lifetime, the field of science was in its infancy and under assault from the Roman Catholic Church when it conflicted with matters of dogma, as in the case of heliocentrism, which conflicted with the Church's model that the earth was at the center of everything.

It was during Descartes' lifetime that Galileo was found by the Inquisition to be suspect for holding scientific ideas contrary to Holy Scripture. Galileo's books were banned, and it was forbidden to publish any of his writings, and also anything he might write in the future. He was placed under house arrest and remained there until he died nine years later in 1642.

This was the intellectual climate Descartes had to deal with.

Descartes put forth the idea that reality is divided into two realms: *res extensa*, the material world or matter – that which has weight and mass; and *res cogitans,* the subjective world of thought – that which has no weight or heft.

In Descartes' view, any expression of matter was worthy of scientific inquiry. He hoped that this division would mollify the Church and temper its view that science was a threat to the order of things. While it can be argued that this did ease some of the tension between religion and science, it is also worth noting that Descartes moved a total of 24 times during his lifetime, searching for a place where he could live and think without fear of reprisal. Of necessity, he was our first free-range philosopher.

Unfortunately, Cartesian dualism's splitting of reality into separate worlds of mind and matter also had an unintentional side effect. For most of the last 300 years science has largely ignored the challenge of investigating how elements of the physical world manifest in the mental world,

and how mental constructs affect the physical. Those who did have the temerity to investigate were ignored at best or ridiculed at worst.

One such exploration into the mind manifesting into the matter happened at the University of Pittsburgh in a pilot study to see if mindfulness meditation could positively affect older adults with chronic low back pain (Morone et al. 2008).

Mindfulness meditation means non-judgmentally paying attention to the present moment. This is done to silence the constant chattering of thoughts in the brain – what is referred to as the monkey mind, or puppy mind, as it were. One of the simplest forms of mindfulness meditation is to focus on one's breathing while repeating the thought: "Breathing in, I know I am breathing in. Breathing out, I know I am breathing out." Every time one's thoughts begin to wander, one refocuses on breathing and returns to the phrase.

The idea is to get to a state of calm, where even if you are aware of random thoughts you are just observing them. So, you may still have the thought, but the thought does not have you.

The results of the study showed in every case that the participants had a decrease in their perception of low back pain. What makes the study disappointing is that it started with 89 participants but only eight made it to the finish line. It was hardly a big enough number to be representative of the overall population. Still, that relatively low number should not cause us to dismiss the results out of hand either.

Meditation has been shown to increase the level of nitric oxide in the body (Kim et al. 2005). Nitric oxide, specifically the nitric oxide donator glyceryl trinitrate, induces relaxation in the fascia (Schleip et al. 2006). And now that we understand the importance of the thoracolumbar fascia as a structure of the low back and the physical fascial connections between the suboccipital muscles and the dural tube (see Chapters 3 and 4), the correlations here should be apparent. Certainly, this merits further investigation with larger numbers.

That investigation happened with a robust sample size of 282, enough to have a randomized clinical trial. The experimental group received the mindfulness training, the control group an educational program based on the 10 Keys to Healthy Aging (Newman et al. 2010). While the results showed improvement in mechanical function, it was short-lived; when surveyed 6 months later those who continued their mindfulness practices sustained a clinically significant (30 per cent) overall improvement in pain intensity (Morone et al. 2016).

Another example, albeit completely anecdotal, of these kinds of phenomena are incidents involving somatoemotional releases (SERs). SERs occur when a change or release of mechanical tension in the body coincides with an emotional response, very often anger or sorrow. While SERs do often, but not always, occur with patients actively suffering from post-traumatic stress disorder (PTSD), many clinicians will report observing SERs in patients who are not diagnosed with PTSD. In fact, I have had this happen to me.

It involved a very distinct memory of a life-threatening event where I nearly strangled to death. I was certainly very afraid that would happen. Psychologically speaking, I had processed that event a long time ago. I was somewhere between the age of four or five when the event happened, but I was in my mid-forties when the SER occurred.

I was at a continuing education seminar and a trusted colleague was performing a fascial release on my left anterior scalene. Rather suddenly I had a distinctive physical – emotional recall of the traumatic event with a level of graphic detail much more vivid than simple recollection. It was as if I was feeling the rope around my neck all over again, and I simultaneously tensed against it, increased my respiration, and began to form tears. It is important to note that my colleague was using an appropriate amount of pressure and in no way did I feel any sense of danger or fear of physical harm during her treatment. Indeed, I also simultaneously felt a sense of deep relief that this part of me was being touched, finally! And following the treatment there was a deeper sense of relief that extended beyond the physical.

It would be wrong to ignore phenomena like these because they fall on the wrong side of Cartesian duality. Phenomena such as these sit there at the intersection of mind and matter, quietly waiting to be investigated. Both Peter Levine and Bessel van der Kolk have been pioneers in this field, often recommending practices such as yoga and interventions like Eye Movement Desensitization and Reprocessing (EMDR) and structural integration.

We have seen in Chapter 4 how the fascial system interacts with the nervous system, but are there other connections between the body and the brain? Might fascia be the conduit for the mind–body connection?

The obvious anatomical structures are the meninges: the dura mater, arachnoid, and the delicate, mesh-like membrane of the pia mater. Rather like our musculoskeletal fascia, the pia follows along all the contours of the brain, all the way to the ependyma where cerebrospinal fluid is produced. The main components of the pia are reticular fibers and, predominantly, collagen. Likewise, the tissue of the dura actually invests all the nerves.

In the microscopic world, there is a uni-directionally arranged fibrous network in the pia, potentially contributing tensile forces throughout the spinal meninges (Nam et al. 2014). Back in the macro world there also appears to be a relation-ship between collagen laxity and anxiety (Bulbena et al. 2006). A more recent study (Michalak et al. 2021) showed that people diagnosed with Major Depressive Disorder (MDD) exhibited heightened stiffness and reduced elasticity in their myofascial tissue. Could there be a natural level of pre-tension in the brain that promotes optimal functioning?

It is also worth noting that collagen is a semi-conductor. Under the right circumstances invol-ving both heat and hydration, the collagen in the body is capable of carrying an electric charge (Tomaselli & Shamos 1974). Some have specu-lated that this quality combined with colla-gen's liquid crystal molecular structure makes it possible for the collagen network to function like a transistor circuit, potentially storing and transmitting information like the microproces-sors in our computers (Oschman 2000).

In the field of nanotechnology, collagen-like triple helix proteins are being used to fabricate nanowires (Hanying 2011), and the University of Tel Aviv has been successfully crafting biode-gradable transistors out of self-assembling blood, milk, and mucus (Hunka 2012). They have not yet tried to do this with collagen (Hunka 2015).

Intriguing as these speculations are, to really explore the possibility of fascia as the conduit of the mind–body connection, we must also take a closer look to a specific class of brain cell called glia. And, perhaps not surprisingly, the story of glia has some curious parallels to the story of fascia.

Neuroscience at the turn of the twentieth century

Santiago Ramón y Cajal was the foremost neuroscientist of the twentieth century. He stud-ied both animal and human brains, looking for patterns in the architecture that would reveal how the brain functions. In the early 1900s he utilized the latest staining methods, producing meticulous illustrations of the cellular parts of the brain, espe-cially neurons (Figure 5.1). His contribution in this regard was easily on a par with that of Vesalius.

Ramón y Cajal created the "neuron doctrine," which established that the brain and nerv-ous system tissues were made of discrete cells, with the neuron as the primary cell. The neu-ron doctrine furthermore clarifies that while neurons are not a continuous, hardwired network, they nonetheless communicate with each other via synapses across spaces called gap junctions. The neuron doctrine asserts that all information exchange and communication in the central nervous system takes place this way.

This was in direct competition with Camillo Golgi's competing reticular theory, which asserted that all the cells in the brain and nerv-ous system were connected like a net, and func-tioned together fluidly.

In 1906, Ramón y Cajal won the Nobel Prize for his work, and the neuron doctrine estab-lished itself at the heart of neuroscience where it remains to this day. Ironically, that same day Golgi would also win a Nobel Prize for creating the staining technique that Ramón y Cajal used, and later modified, to explore brain cells and develop the neuron doctrine.

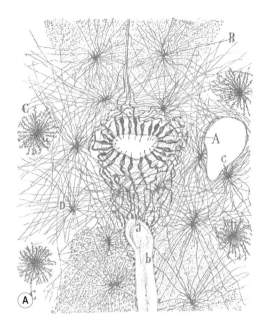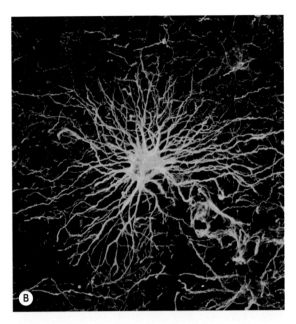

Figure 5.1
(A) Drawing of neuroglia (denoted by C) by Ramón y Cajal. Compare this to actual neuroglia (B).
(A) Courtesy of Wellcome Library, London. (B) Reproduced with kind permission from Maiken Nedergaard.

While neurons were not the only cells in the brain, it was generally accepted that they were the most important cells in the brain because they were larger, and their axons covered longer distances than those of other nerve cells. So, they were bigger, longer, and had processes that looked like tree branches; however, neurons were outnumbered by a much smaller cell. These cells were initially given the name "spider cells" by Ramón y Cajal because of their shape. They were later given the name "glia," which is Greek for "glue."

These spider cells were estimated to outnumber neurons by nine to one on average. That is nine glia for each neuron. Remember that old saying that you only use 10 per cent of the brain? This is where I think that saying came from.

Although in a recent interview astrophysicist Neil deGrasse Tyson said this idea was a misinterpretation of something someone who studied brain damage had said in the early 1900s. This scientist was of the opinion that the brain is so complex that we really only understand about 10 per cent of how it works. This was mistakenly repeated over and over again as "we only use 10 per cent of our brain." Perhaps this is another case of "both/and."

As recently as 2014 it was stated that glia comprises 85 per cent of brain cells (Fields 2014), and many neuroscience textbooks and popular articles continue to make the claim that there can be anywhere from 10 to 50 times more glia than neurons. This is considered controversial by some. In her book *Medical Neurobiology* (2017),

Peggy Mason says "there are roughly as many glial cells as there are neurons." That idea is well-reinforced by Suzana Herculano-Houzel (2014) who proposes a 1:1 ratio and no single uniform variations in that ratio relative to brain size. She has found evidence for an increased glia-to-neuron ratio based on increased neuron size, however. Some dismiss her findings as she does not employ more traditional, and tediously time-consuming, cell counting methods. An excellent overview of the history of brain cell counting and the employment of newer methods was published by von Bartheld et al. in 2016. He also comes down squarely on the 1:1 side of things, although he did find a higher glia-to-neuron ratio in primates, but in the spinal cord rather than in the brain (Bahney & von Bartheld 2018). Other fascinating variations in this ratio exist, and as the body doesn't tend to grow extra parts there must be some significance to these differences, as there is in the fact that glia and neurons do communicate.

Meanwhile, back in the nineteenth century, the idea that glia and neurons were somehow able to signal to each other was first proposed by Carl Ludwig Schleich in 1894. It was quickly dismissed and forgotten. Instead, the idea was put forth that the glia were just nerve putty, organic packing peanuts that, like fascia, held the brain together, and in this case also served to insulate the neurons. To be fair, Ramón y Cajal was not too sure about this, but when his brother and fellow researcher Pedro got on board with the idea, he relented and adopted this theory about glia for himself.

What is curious to note is that even in those days they knew that the more sophisticated the life form, the greater the overall number of glia. Even with that knowledge there was no real effort made to study the glia. As far as the neuroscientists of the time were concerned, neurons were the obvious stars, standing out like celebrities in a crowd of adoring glia. Obviously, from what could be seen neurons had to be more important. But what we see and what it actually means are not always that obvious.

It turns out that Schleich was right – glia and neurons *do* communicate with each other. Furthermore, glia respond to neurotransmitters and even regulate which neurons fire, and more.

If the brain is a vast orchestra, then the glia may well conduct the symphony that is played by the neurons. But these discoveries, which are still not widely known, would take more than 100 years to come to light.

Neuroscience at the dawn of the twenty-first century

In the late 1980s it was first discovered that the neurotransmitter glutamate could trigger a calcium cascade in glial cells (Figure 5.2) (Cornell-Bell et al. 1990). This was a big deal because up to that point glia were thought to be completely inert. This suggested that there could be a long-range signaling system within the brain. Four years later, Maiken Nedergaard confirmed the existence of this signaling network in a type of glia known as astrocytes (Nedergaard 1994).

A few years after that, near the turn of the century, a researcher at the National Institute for Health, R. Douglas Fields, was carrying out imaging experiments with a live culture of dorsal root ganglion (DRG) neurons. The DRG neurons were electrically stimulated so that calcium would flow into the cell. Using a special dye, this process could be seen and mapped. It worked flawlessly every time.

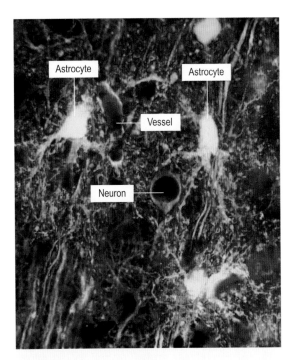

Figure 5.2
Astrocyte calcium signaling.
Reproduced with kind permission from Maiken Nedergaard.

In the interest of being thorough, Fields had glial cells, specifically Schwann cells, added to the culture. In the peripheral nervous system, Schwann cells attach to the long axon of the neuron and also form myelin, the insulation around the nerve. It was generally assumed that the Schwann cells could not detect neuronal activity any more than the plastic coating around a wire can feel electricity. Schwann cells were inert, weren't they? Just because astroglia were shown not to be inert did not mean that was the case for all glia cells.

So, the experiment was repeated, this time with the addition of the Schwann cells and that is exactly what happened. Nothing happened for the first 15 seconds. Then, one by one, the glia began to light up brilliantly, signaling that they too had detected the signal and then they started increasing their own stores of calcium. Somehow the glia had detected the calcium change in the nearby neurons and responded accordingly (Fields 2004). Even though he did not yet understand everything this might mean, obviously, it was still a significant moment:

I just wish I could get across the amazement of that finding...that these cells that were thought to be stuffing between neurons were communicating. (Fields 2009)

While neuroscientists were initially and understandably wary of hitching a ride on the glia bandwagon, glia research has exploded in the last decade and it is turning out to be quite important.

Meet the glia

Because glia are often referred to as, and are too often considered to function like, the connective tissue of the brain, one might understandably think they are part of the fascial web, but as far as we know they are not (Figure 5.3). Most glia are derived from the same embryonic layer as the nervous system – the ectoderm. The exception is microglia, which develop in the same layer as the rest of the connective tissue matrix – the mesoderm.

The human brain contains more than 100 trillion synaptic connections, which form all the neural circuitry of the brain. But the brain, and thereby thinking, is in fact electrochemical in nature. Glia cells are essential to the formation of healthy synapses and the long-term survival of neurons (Smith 1998). Glia can sense neural activity, send messages, and regulate synaptic activity between neurons (Eroglu & Barnes 2010).

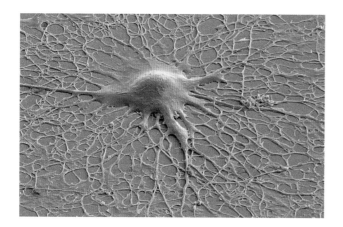

Figure 5.3
A human glia cell sitting in the neural net, looking suspiciously like a fibroblast in the fascial net.
Reproduced with kind permission from Tom Deerinck.

Glia have the same neurotransmitter cell receptor sites as neurons do. This enables them to listen to neurons by picking up on the neurotransmitters they produce. The glia can then send chemical messages, via calcium waves through potassium ion channels, to glia in other parts of the brain. These glia, in turn, can produce the same neurotransmitters – in essence, they can talk to the neurons in that area even though those neurons have no direct synaptic pathway with the neuron that originated the signal (Fields 2004).

To put it another way, neurons and synapses behave like old-style telephone networks. There needs to be a direct series of wires between my phone and yours in order for us to communicate with each other. Glia are like cell phones; they can call everyone they have a number for, and they can call into the old-school telephones as well. In this respect, they are remarkably similar to sensory nerves.

The emerging science of glia is changing views on how the brain works and pointing to new directions for the treatment of mental illnesses and conditions such as Parkinson's and amyotrophic lateral sclerosis (ALS) (Yeager 2015).

Glia also have a relationship with chronic and neuropathic pain (Fields 2009, Milligan & Watkins 2009). Significantly, while glia both release and help to maintain anti-inflammatory factors, prolonged exposure to opioids will cause glia to release proinflammatory cytokines (Johnston et al. 2004).

Like the fibroblast network, the glia form another non-neuronal, mechanosensitive network in the body. There are four principal types of glia. Some sources will, confusingly, only list three of the four, and, more confusing still, not always the same three types. The three types of glia that exist throughout the central nervous system are oligodendrocytes, microglia, and astrocytes. The other type of glia, the Schwann cells, exists only in the peripheral nervous system.

We will meet them in that order.

Oligodendrocytes

Oligodendrocytes are found everywhere throughout the central nervous system (CNS) (Figure 5.4). These "stubby dendrites" (hence the name) have many long processes that are responsible for generating myelin sheaths around axons.

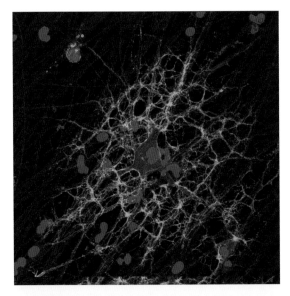

Figure 5.4
Oligodendrocyte tendrils (green) respond to glutamate released by active axons (purple) ramping up the local production of myelin.
Image reproduced with kind permission from R. Douglas Fields and Hiroaki Wake, NIH.

respond to supply and demand. In the symphony of the brain, oligodendrocytes are the rhythm section.

It is speculated that oligodendrocytes help the brain to continuously adapt to incoming information. They are essential in synchronizing neuronal firing in different parts of the brain, where a delay of even a millisecond could cause a failure in coordination (Pajevic et al. 2014). It is thought the impairment of activity-dependent myelination could be a contributing factor to conditions such as dyslexia, epilepsy, and schizophrenia.

Microglia

Microglia (Figure 5.5), the only glia to derive from the mesoderm, differentiate in the bone marrow. This is only natural as microglia serve as the immune system of the brain and central nervous system. There is approximately one microglia for every neuron, so it is as if each neuron comes with its own bodyguard.

Myelin, as you may recall, is a lipid-protein that insulates the neuronal axons so that they may conduct their interneuronal communication with more efficiency – just like the coating on an electrical wire improves the flow of electricity and keeps the electrons from leaking out. Recent discoveries of how the myelin is actually laid out, with varying degrees of thickness within the same axon, seem to have long-term implications for neuronal communication and brain development. MRI studies involving children learning piano and adults learning juggling showed actual structural change to myelin in the brain (Scholz et al. 2009). This process is referred to as activity-dependent myelination.

So, it seems that in learning complex, coordinated neuromuscular activity, oligodendrocytes

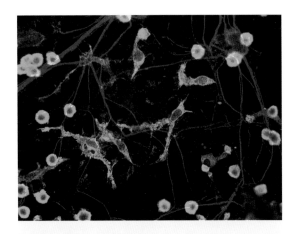

Figure 5.5
Microglia – the immune cell in the glia network.
Image courtesy of Gerry Shaw (https://creativecommons.org/licenses/by-sa/3.0/legalcode).

Microglia also display intriguing morphological qualities. They are curiously plastic, adapting their shape to the cellular terrain around them. While it is amusing to see a parallel between that behavior and the way fibroblasts align with the fiber direction of the underlying collagen substrate, in fact most neuroscientists speculate that microglia do this as a form of cellular camouflage – all the better to lie in wait for potential cellular attackers. In fact, microglia are so good at blending in with the cellular scenery that up until the mid-1990s scientists debated about whether or not they actually existed!

One thing we do know is that when they sense injury or infection, these normally docile and solitary cells turn into highly mobile ameboid cells, springing into action to repel and destroy the cellular invasion. In another parallel, it is intriguing that the integrins of the microglia seem to be involved in creating this motion, and, along with various cytokines, one of the main substances that microglia produce during the immune response phase is nitric oxide (Maruyama et al. 2012).

Recent evidence also points to the role of microglia in Alzheimer's disease, although the exact nature of their role is still being debated. It is agreed that the prominence of microglia in places where the brain has been damaged by Alzheimer's is not coincidental, but the exact nature of microglia involvement remains elusive (Landhuis 2016). Some experiments seem to indicate that microglia exacerbate the problem; however, other studies indicate it may be chronic inflammation that prevents microglia from doing their job effectively (Guillot-Sestier et al. 2015) and researchers are looking for ways to restore glia to their proper health.

Astrocytes

Astrocytes (Figure 5.6) are so named for their star-like shape, aesthetically a much more appealing name than Ramón y Cajal's "spider cells." Astrocytes are the most abundant glial cell in the body, with a glia-to-neuron ratio of anywhere from two to ten astrocytes per neuron depending on the area of the brain. Some researchers theorize that there may be as many different types of astrocytes as there are neurons, which accounts for some sources listing seven or more types of glia, but for the time being the scientific consensus gives them all the same classification.

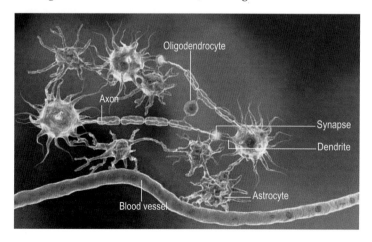

Figure 5.6

Glia and neurons working together. Here we see five astrocytes in the neighborhood of three neurons. Also, note the oligodendrocyte providing the myelin to insulate the axon. Oligodendrocytes are in this way similar to Schwann cells in the peripheral nervous system.

Reproduced with kind permission from Jeff Johnson, Hybrid Medical Animations.

Astrocytes literally support neurons by providing a physical matrix for structural support (hence the "fascia of the brain" analogy). Just like neurons and fibroblasts, astrocytes form an interconnected, multicellular network via their gap junctions. It is in these gap junctions that astrocytes perform their custodial duties.

Neurons require a very precise environment in order to fire properly. If ion imbalances sufficiently pollute the environment, the neuron will fall silent, unable to fire. Astrocytes remove excess potassium ions from the cellular environment of the brain, the excess potassium being a cellular by-product of neuronal firing. This enables the neuron to maintain its proper electrical charge.

Astrocytes clean up the mess, enabling neurons to function properly, but they are more than janitors. They perform triage, forming scar tissue during brain injury. They also regulate breathing and have huge implications in the process of how we learn.

While there has long been the belief that a certain class of neurons regulates breathing, they have yet to be found. What have been found are astrocytes in the medulla oblongata that respond to decreases in pH by increasing respiration (Gourine et al. 2010). Exercise is one example as it causes the body to produce more carbon dioxide than normal, which drops the pH levels. Astrocytes in the medulla oblongata respond to this change in pH by producing ATP to increase the rate of respiration.

The astrocytes' role in learning is a bit more complex.

Astrocytes both discriminate and integrate the flow of information between the synapses.

Specifically, astrocytes found in the cerebral cortex have all the necessary physical, chemical, and structural components to process and integrate sensory experiences. They also contain all the neurotransmitters associated with consciousness. Since there is no one specific anatomical region of the brain that integrates sensory information, it has been further hypothesized that the protoplasmic astrocytes form a syncytium that is responsible for what we recognize as consciousness (Robertson 2002).

Astroglia also produce many of the neurotransmitters associated with so-called muscle memory – the ability of the body, over time, to remember how to physically perform tasks without the need to consciously think about it. Like driving home after work, doing a series of sun salutes, or performing a piece of music. No-one is really sure how muscle memory actually works or what the precise mechanisms are, but we do know it requires significant brain activity in many areas, including the prefrontal cortex, primary motor cortex, cerebellum, and the anterior cingulate gyrus.

A model has been created to show how astrocytes can both inhibit and stimulate certain synaptic pathways (via ATP, glutamate, and other neurotransmitters) to affect the patterns, speed, and modulation of physical tasks and are thereby essential to the formation of muscle memory (Hassanpoor 2012).

More than just a theory, the role of glia in intelligence and neuromuscular coordination may have been proven in the labs at the University of Rochester Medical Center, New York.

As we have mentioned earlier, the number of glia in general, and astrocytes specifically, increase exponentially with increases in the sophistication and intelligence of the life form. What is also interesting to note is that the size and speed of astroglia change as we progress up the evolutionary ladder.

For example, human astrocytes are 2.6 times larger and ten times longer than mouse astrocytes. And the calcium waves travel five times faster through our brains than in rodent brains. We also have additional types of astrocytes, including interlaminar astrocytes that have long fibers that extend through the cortex into the parts of the brain involving learning, memory, and creativity (Oberheim et al. 2009).

In an experiment that appears to have been inspired by Daniel Keyes's *Flowers for Algernon*, human glia progenitor cells were transplanted into the brains of mice to see if they would change the way the brains work. They did. The mice became smarter.

Over a period of several months, the speed of calcium transmissions increased threefold and neuron-to-neuron communication was enhanced. Moreover, in simple tasks of memorization and learning, the human glia-enhanced mice consistently outperformed the control group of normal mice with normal mouse brains (Han et al. 2013). This kind of "brain-doping" does, however, disqualify the mice from participating in the annual Mice Olympics.

Other interesting astrocyte findings go back to the 1930s and Hungarian psychopathologist Ladislas von Meduna. He discovered a noticeable lack of astrocytes in the cerebral cortex of people suffering from both schizophrenia and depression; whereas people who suffered from epileptic seizures had an unusually high astrocyte count (Yuhas 2012).

They kept Einstein's brain

It is a well-known story that when Albert Einstein died in 1955 his brain was stolen by Thomas Harvey. The story only seems to get more colorful as time goes by. What we can definitely say is this: Harvey was the pathologist who conducted the autopsy on Einstein and he took an extensive series of photographs of Einstein's brain. He also kept it in a jar in a cardboard box under his desk.

He believed it was his duty to keep the brain he preserved for study, so that the world's leading neuroscientists could find out what made Einstein, well, such an Einstein. He also believed he had the permission to do this. Apparently somewhere down the line Albert had said it was okay to study his body after he was gone, but Einstein's family disagreed. Harvey lost his job at Princeton, but somehow managed to keep the brain.

Over the next three decades, Harvey would parcel out pieces to researchers throughout the world. One of them was Marian Diamond, professor of anatomy at the University of California, Berkeley.

While we know that Einstein's brain was smaller than average, it also had some striking topographic differences, with asymmetrical parietal lobes and a prominent "knob" in the somatosensory cortex associated with the left hand – a feature not at all unusual in musicians, and Einstein was a prodigious violinist (Falk et al. 2013, Costandi 2012).

Marian Diamond had a different idea. She wanted to look at the glia-to-neuron ratio of Einstein's brain. She was aware of early epigenetic studies at Purdue showing that rats living in stimulating, experience-rich environments have more glia per neuron than rats living in impoverished conditions (Diamond 1999). Since glial cells are capable of multiplying throughout one's life, Diamond reasoned that more active neurons would need a greater number of support cells than those that were less active. She also reasoned that the more highly evolved areas of the brain would have a higher glia-to-neuron ratio.

Remember, at this time the notion of glial communication was not even thought about, but nonetheless Diamond respected the importance of glia, and it was obvious to her that glia responded to supply and demand.

Diamond collected small, sugar-cube-sized pieces of brain from the right and left prefrontal cortex and inferior parietal cortex from 11 male brains to use as her control group. These areas were chosen because of their association with higher brain functions. She then began to pester Thomas Harvey.

After three years of calling Harvey about once every six months, a package arrived for Diamond at the university. Floating in an alcohol solution inside a mayonnaise jar were the four sugar-cube-sized pieces of Einstein's brain she had been asking for. They were from the same areas of the brain as her control samples. Fortunately, the pieces of Einstein's brain had been embedded in celloidin, which hardens like plastic, and this made them ideal for Diamond's study, because she would have to make slices of about 6 microns (or six-thousandths of a millimeter) in length.

While Diamond found higher glia-to-neuron ratios than average in all the samples of Einstein's brain, she did not consider them statistically big enough to be significant, except in the left inferior parietal area.

The left inferior parietal lobule is a very important place in the brain. It is the confluence of the auditory, visual, and somatosensory cortexes, and is thought to be one of the areas where multiple modes of information are processed and integrated. It is widely regarded to be the area of the brain for conceptual and abstract thinking. In this area, Einstein's brain had nearly twice as many astrocytes than the average brain (Diamond et al. 1985, Diamond 1999).

Schwann cells

The only glia to exist outside of the brain and central nervous system are the Schwann cells. The Schwann cells abide in the peripheral nervous system. They are very dynamic cells and will undergo cell division in response to injuries in the peripheral nerves. They are considered the regulators of nerve development (Mirsky et al. 2002). Like the rest of the glia, Schwann cells were largely not regarded as having any influence on the nervous system, although that idea evaporated in light of the calcium induction experiments of R. Douglas Fields, as highlighted earlier in this chapter.

There are three distinct types of Schwann cells: myelinating, nonmyelinating, and perisynaptic (also referred to as terminal). Curiously, each type of Schwann cell has a different structure and function. One could argue that they should be considered as three different cell types although they do share a common ancestor – the neural crest cell.

Myelinating Schwann cells

The myelinating Schwann cells cover the entire length of the nerve fibers like tiny beads of dew, stopping where the fibers enter the spinal cord. They cover only large-diameter axons (known for their very fast transmission times). They are, obviously, in charge of nerve myelination, and also of remyelination of damaged nerves in the peripheral nervous system (PNS).

Myelinating Schwann cells have been transplanted from the PNS directly into the spine of rats with damaged spinal cords. Since the rats' own cells were used, there was little possibility of rejection of the transplant. A systematic review of 13 trials comprising 283 rats has shown that Schwann cell transplants can significantly improve locomotor recovery regardless of dosage; in this case, the dose would be the actual number of transplanted cells (Yang et al. 2015). The Miami Project to Cure Paralysis is currently working to see if Schwann cell transplants can work the same way in humans.

Nonmyelinating Schwann cells

Nonmyelinating Schwann cells have great globular shapes. Some refer to them as "fist-like" in the way they seem to grasp slender, small-diameter axons into protective bundles by secreting cytoplasm from their own membrane. In this case, they do act like packing peanuts to protect the nonmyelinated nerves.

If myelination is so good at improving efficiency, why aren't all axons myelinated? Good question. The simple answer is that not all nerves need to be that fast.

First, not all axons have to cover great distances. And second, not all neurons have to be fast to do their job correctly. These are the C-fiber axons, which mostly carry certain kinds of sensory information, such as the C-fiber axons sending me the message about a dull ache in my right hip (most likely caused by my spending the last several hours sitting and writing). That information does not need to travel so fast. It is necessary but not urgent.

Now when I get up to make a nice cup of tea and stretch a little, and I nearly spill scalding tea on myself, but avoid doing so, that information has to travel fast so the nerves transmitting those signals will send them along myelinated channels.

Perisynaptic (terminal) Schwann cells

The final, and most "fascia-nating," Schwann cell is the perisynaptic Schwann cell (PSC) whose domain is in the neuromuscular junction (Figure 5.7), where the motor commands of the nervous system are carried out. The neuromuscular junction is considered a highly plastic area because of its ability to adapt to constant change and respond to injury. PSCs are a vital component of this synaptic plasticity (Ko & Robitaille 2015).

As highlighted in the previous chapter, the neuromuscular junction is where Golgi tendon organs and Pacini receptors relay messages of tension and vibration throughout the fascial net. It is here that the terminal endings of the fascial mechanoreceptors are wrapped by the PSCs (which is why they are often called "terminal" Schwann cells). They are vital to short-term plasticity at the neuromuscular junction (Colomar & Robitaille 2004).

Nerve resection studies have also shown that the PSCs are vital to the early development of fascial mechanoreceptors. In cases where they have been removed during early stages of life, the Golgi and Pacini receptors do not form correctly,

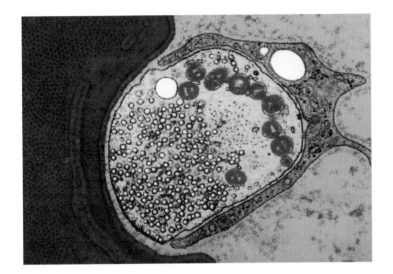

Figure 5.7
A Schwann cell (green) encloses a nerve terminal (blue) with muscle fiber (red). Photograph by D. Fawcett.
Reproduced with kind permission from Science Source.

or at all, nor do they regenerate after injury. While it is possible for a nerve to communicate with muscle without the presence of PSCs, these connections are considered transient. It seems that perisynaptic Schwann cells are necessary to keep mechanoreceptors alive and that they have an interdependent relationship (Kopp et al. 1997).

This architectural relationship cannot be random. Nature as a rule follows patterns and likes to conserve energy, so it is logical to assume this arrangement of glia, mechanoreceptors, and fascia has some implicate order. In the same way that glia listen to and influence the neurons, are Schwann cells influenced by the Golgi tendon organs and Pacini corpuscles and vice versa? To the best of my knowledge, this area of potential fascia – glia crossover is a wide-open area for study, with no significant research currently being carried out (Fields 2012).

Like fascia science, glia science is still in its early days. Very often I come back to this quote from R. Douglas Fields, and reflect how sonorously it resonates with what we say about fascia:

When you see an egret take flight, soaring with grace from a marshy shore, or a stallion galloping in an open field, you are seeing what glia have enabled vertebrates to accomplish: swiftness and grace of motion.

References

Bahney J and von Bartheld C S (2018) The cellular composition and glia-neuron ratio in the spinal cord of a human and a non-human primate: Comparison with other species and brain regions. Anat Rec (Hoboken). April; 301 (4) 697–710.

Bulbena A, Gago J, Sperry L and Bergé D (2006) The relationship between frequency and intensity of fears and a collagen condition. Depress Anxiety. July; 23 (7) 412–417.

Colomar A and Robitaille R (2004) Glial modulation of synaptic transmission at the neuromuscular junction. Glia. August; 47 (3) 284–289.

Cornell-Bell A H, Finkbeiner S M, Cooper M S and Smith S J (1990) Glutamate induces calcium waves in cultured astrocytes: Long-range glial signaling. Science. January; 247 (4941) 470–473.

Costandi M (2012) Snapshots explore Einstein's unusual brain. Nature: News. November 16, 2012. Available: www.nature.com/articles/nature.2012.11836 [May 18, 2022].

Diamond M C (1999) Why Einstein's brain? Lecture given at Doe Library, January 8, 1999. Transcription available: https://web.archive.org/web/20170504015541/http://education.jhu.edu/PD/newhorizons/Neurosciences/articles/einstein/index.html [May 23, 2022].

Diamond M C, Scheibel A B, Murphy G M Jr. and Harvey T (1985) On the brain of a scientist: Albert Einstein. Exp Neurol. April; 88 (1) 198–204.

Eroglu C and Barnes B A (2010) Regulation of synaptic activity by glia. Nature. November; 468 (7321) 223–231.

Falk D, Lepore F E and Noe A (2013) The cerebral cortex of Albert Einstein: A description and preliminary analysis of unpublished photographs. Brain. April; 136 (4) 1304–1327.

Fields R D (2004) The other half of the brain. Scientific American. April; 290 (4) 54–61.

Fields R D (2009) New culprits in chronic pain. Scientific American. November; 301 (5) 50–57.

Fields R D (2012) Correspondence with the author.

Fields R D (2014) Myelin—more than insulation. Science. April; 344 (6181) 264–266.

Gourine A V, Kasymov V, Marina N et al. (2010) Astrocytes control breathing through pH-dependent release of ATP. Science. July; 329 (5991) 571–575.

Guillot-Sestier M V, Doty K R and Town T (2015) Innate immunity fights Alzheimer's disease. Trends Neurosci. November; 38 (11) 674–681.

Han X, Chen M, Fushun W et al. (2013) Forebrain engraftment by human glial progenitor cells enhances synaptic plasticity and learning in adult mice. Cell Stem Cell. March; 12 (3) 342–353.

Hanying B (2011) Genetically modified collagen-like triple helix protein as biomimetic template to fabricate metal/semiconductor nanowires. Dissertation, City University of New York, 121 pages; 3443928.

Hassanpoor H, Fallah A and Raza M (2012) New role for astroglia in learning: Formation of muscle memory. Med Hypothesis. December; 79 (6) 770–773.

Herculano-Houzel S (2014) The glia/neuron ratio: How it varies uniformly across brain structure and species and what that means for brain physiology and evolution. Glia. September; 62 (9) 1377–1391.

Hunka G (2012) Biodegradable transistors – made from us. Public Release. American Friends of Tel Aviv University. EurekaAlert! Available: www.eurekalert.org/pub_releases/2012-03/afot-bt-030712.php [May 18, 2022].

Hunka G (2015) Email correspondence with author.

Johnston I N, Milligan E D, Wieseler-Frank J et al. (2004) A role for proinflammatory cytokines and fractalkine in analgesia, tolerance and subsequent pain facilitation induced by chronic intrathecal morphine. J Neurosci. August; 24 (33) 7353–7365.

Kim D H, Moon Y S, Kim H S et al. (2005) Effect of Zen Meditation on serum nitric oxide activity and lipid peroxidation. Prog Neuropsychopharmacol Biol Psychiatry. February; 29 (2) 327–331.

Ko C P and Robitaille R (2015) Perisynaptic Schwann cells at the neuromuscular synapse: Adaptable, multitasking glial cells. Cold Spring Harb Perspect Biol. August; 7 (10) a020503.

Kopp D M, Trachtenberg J T and Thompson W J (1997) Glial growth factor rescues Schwann cells of mechanoreceptors from denervation-induced apoptosis. J Neurosci. September; 17 (17) 6697–6706.

Landhuis E (2016) Uncovering new players in the fight against Alzheimer's. Scientific American, Neuroscience blog. April. Available: www.scientificamerican.com/article/uncovering-new-players-in-the-fight-against-alzheimer-s [May 18, 2022].

Maruyama K, Okamoto T and Shimaoka M (2012) Integrins and nitric oxide in the regulation of glia cells: Potential roles in pathological pain. J Anesth Clin Res. June; 4, 2; doi:10.4172/2155-6148.1000292.

Mason P (2017) Medical Neurobiology, 2nd edn. Oxford: Oxford University Press, p. 17.

Michalak J, Aranmolate L, Bon A et al. (2021) Myofascial tissue and depression. Cognit Ther Res. December; 1–13. doi: 10.1007/s10608-021-10282-w. [Epub ahead of print].

Milligan E D and Watkins L R (2009) Pathological and protective roles of glia in chronic pain. Nat Rev Neurosci. January; 10 (1) 23–36.

Mirsky R, Jessen K R, Brennan A et al. (2002) Schwann Cells as regulators of nerve development. J Physiol Paris. January–March; 96 (1–2) 17–24.

Morone N E, Greco C M, Moore C G et al. (2016) A mind-body program for older adults with chronic low back pain. A randomized clinical trial. JAMA Intern Med. March; 176 (3) 329–337.

Morone N E, Greco C M and Weiner D K (2008) Mindfulness meditation for the treatment of chronic low back pain in older adults: A randomized controlled pilot study. Pain. February; 134 (3) 310–319.

Nam M H, Baek M, Lim J et al. (2014) Discovery of a novel fibrous tissue in the spinal pia mater by polarized light microscopy. Connect Tissue Res. April; 55 (2) 147–155.

Nedergaard M (1994) Direct signaling from astrocytes to neurons in cultures of mammalian brain cells. Science. March; 263 (5154) 1768–1771.

Newman A B, Bayles C M, Milas C N et al. (2010) The 10 Keys to Healthy Aging: Findings from an innovative program in the community. J Aging Health. August; 22 (5) 547–566.

Oberheim N A, Takano T, Han X et al. (2009) Uniquely hominid features of adult human astrocytes. J Neurosci. March; 29 (10) 3276–3287.

Oschman J L (2000) Energy Medicine: The Scientific Basis. Elsevier, pp. 41–58.

Pajevic S, Basser P J and Fields R D (2014) Role of myelin plasticity in oscillation and synchrony of neuronal activity. Neuroscience. September; 276, 135–147.

Robertson J M (2002) The Astrocentric Hypothesis: Proposed role of astrocytes in consciousness and memory formation. J Physiol Paris. April–June; 96 (3–4) 251–255.

Schleip R, Klingler W and Lehmann-Horn F (2006) Fascia is able to contract in a smooth muscle-like manner and thereby influence musculoskeletal mechanics. J Biomech. 39 (Supplement 1) S488.

Scholz, J, Klein M C, Behrens T E and Johansen-Berg H (2009) Training induces changes in white matter architecture. Nat Neurosci. November; 12 (11) 1370–1371.

Sigman M and Dehaene S (2008) Brain mechanisms of serial and parallel processing during dual-task performance. J Neurosci. July; 28 (30) 7585–7598.

Smith S J (1998) Synapses: Glia help synapses form and function. Current Biology. 8, R158–R160.

Tomaselli V P and Shamos M H (1974) Electrical properties of hydrated collagen. II. Semiconductor properties. Biopolymers. December; 13 (12) 2423–2434.

von Bartheld C S, Bahney J and Herculano-Houzel S (2016) The search for true numbers of neurons and glial cells in the human brain: A review of 150 years of cell counting. J Comp Neurol. December; 524 (18) 3865–3895.

Yang L, Ge Y, Tang J et al. (2015) Schwann cells transplantation improves locomotor recovery in rat models with spinal cord injury: A systematic review and meta-analysis. Cell Physiol Biochem. December; 37 (6) 2171–2182.

Yeager A (2015) Maestros of learning and memory: Glia prove to be more than the brain's maintenance crew. Science News. August; 188 (4) 19–21.

Yuhas D (2012) Know your Neurons: Meet the Glia. May 18. Available: https://blogs.scientificamerican.com/brainwaves/know-your-neurons-meet-the-glia [May 4, 2022].

Further reading

Armati P J (2007) The Biology of Schwann Cells: Development, Differentiation and Immunomodulation. New York, NY: Cambridge University Press.

Damasio A R (1994) Descartes' Error: Emotion, Reason and the Human Brain. New York, NY: Grosset/Putnam.

Doidge N (2007) The Brain That Changes Itself: Stories of Personal Triumph from the Frontiers of Brain Science. Penguin Life.

Fields R D (2009) The Other Brain: The Scientific and Medical Breakthroughs That Will Heal Our Brains and Revolutionize Our Health. New York, NY: Simon & Schuster.

Koob A (2009) The Root of Thought – Unlocking Glia: The Brain Cell That Will Help Us Sharpen Our Wits, Heal Injury, and Treat Brain Disease. Upper Saddle River, NJ: Pearson Education/FT Press.

Levine P and Frederick A (1997) Waking the Tiger. Berkeley, CA: North Atlantic Books.

Schwartz J M and Begley S (2002) The Mind and the Brain: Neuroplasticity and the Power of Mental Force. New York, NY: Regan Books.

van der Kolk B (2015) The Body Keeps the Score: Brain, Mind, and Body in the Healing of Trauma. New York, NY: Penguin.

Wellnesstalkradio.com (2015) Interview with R. Douglas Fields, "The Other Brain," conducted by Kristin Costello. Available: www.youtube.com/watch?v=m-oLHCS4-Kg [May 18, 2022].

Fascia and the Organs

6

If the cranial brain believes itself surrounded by a knowable world that can be controlled, the brain in our belly is in touch with the world's mystery. The fact that the second brain has been discovered, forgotten, and rediscovered by medicine three times in the past century suggests how complicated our relationship with our bodily intelligence is.

—Amnon Buchbinder

Alimentary, my dear Watson!

The visceral fascia, also referred to as the inner fasciae, is complicated and not because of the basic structure. In fact, the organization of the inner fasciae mirrors the fascial layout of both the nerve and the muscle fasciae. It just seems more complicated because of all the twists and turns.

From beginning to end, the visceral fascia covers the territory from the cranial base to the bottom of the pelvic cavity. Less obliquely, one could also say it connects the mouth to the buttocks. That passage, taken as a whole, is the alimentary canal, but from the fascial perspective we also must include the lungs, heart, and kidneys. They are off-ramps of the alimentary expressway but are still a part of the whole system.

Let's keep mixing metaphors. This chapter is going to be like taking the Paris Batobus. The Batobus floats along the River Seine, giving the big picture of the City of Lights from the perspective of the river that flows down the middle of the city. The Batobus allows passengers to disembark along certain points of the tour

for more exploration. By the end of the journey, you will know more about Paris than you did before, but there are so many streets, neighborhoods, *arrondissements,* cul-de-sacs, and special places, like the roundabout at the Arc de Triomphe (where 12 different avenues converge into a large, multiple-lane traffic circle), that you realize that despite all you have seen you have barely scratched the surface.

This chapter is going to be like that. For those of you wishing for more, I encourage you to use the "tour guides" listed in the References and Further Reading sections. For now, jump on the "boat bus," keep your arms and legs inside at all times, and let's begin!

The basics

The visceral fascia (also known as the inner fasciae or subserous membrane) holds the organs within the body cavity. The organs are wrapped in a double layer of fascia with a sliding layer in between the two (Figure 6.1). The outermost fascial layer is called the parietal layer. The middle part is called the serous membrane and is analogous to a sliding layer of fascia between the muscles. The deepest layer, often referred to

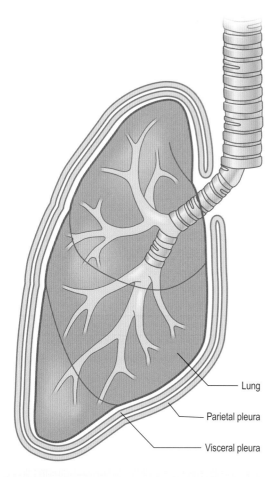

Figure 6.1
The "double-bagged" concept as shown with the lung. The visceral fascia folds in on itself, creating two distinct but completely contiguous "layers."

Lung

Parietal pleura

Visceral pleura

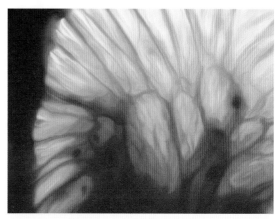

Figure 6.2
Far from being just a fascial bag the mesentery is now considered to be an organ. The mesentery is a fold in the peritoneum which attaches the stomach, small intestine, pancreas, and spleen to the abdomen. When held to the light one can appreciate its complex neurovascular network, necessary for taking nourishment from the intestines to the body.
Photo by Nicole Trombley and Rachelle Clauson. Courtesy of AnatomySCAPES.com.

as the "skin" of the organ, is called the visceral layer. This layer is somewhat analogous to the epimysium that surrounds a muscle. This layer is always given a specific name, such as pericardium to denote the fascial bag around the heart, or mesentery (Figure 6.2) for the layer around the intestines.

Keep in mind that this is all one tissue and it is connected to the rest of the fascial net. In the simplest terms, it is a protective double bag around each organ with a sliding layer in the middle to keep everything lubricated and moving. There are also specialized thickenings in the visceral fascia that are referred to as "ligaments" because they function as ligaments (Figure 6.3). If your liver, for instance, did not have some movement within your body, it would not feel comfortable to bend over, let alone dance.

Visceral fascial tone is important. Too little tone and organs fall out of place or prolapse. If the tone is too tight, it will restrict motility – the natural physiologic motion of the organ – and impede proper function.

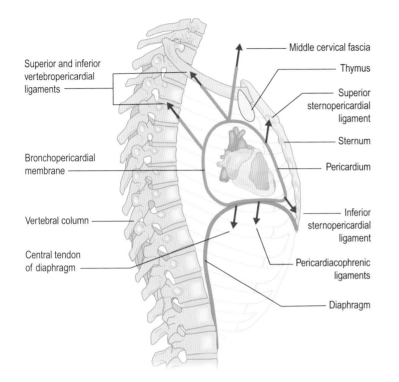

Middle cervical fascia

Thymus

Superior and inferior
vertebropericardial
ligaments

Superior
sternopericardial
ligament

Sternum

Bronchopericardial
membrane

Pericardium

Inferior
sternopericardial
ligament

Vertebral column

Central tendon
of diaphragm

Pericardiacophrenic
ligaments

Diaphragm

Figure 6.3
A sagittal view of the suspensory ligaments of the heart and pericardium. In the van der Wal model (see Chapter 3) these distinctions would be merely topographical, and holistically the ligaments would serve as one very complex dynament.
Modified with permission from Stecco, L. and Stecco, C. (2013) *Fascial Manipulation for Internal Dysfunctions*. Padova, Italy: Piccin Nuova Libraria S.p.A.

While our focus is on the organs, it is also important to note that the inner fasciae also include the fascia that surrounds the glands and the vascular fascial sheaths around arteries, veins, and the adventitia, the fascial covering around blood vessels, which also contain their own fibroblasts and free nerve endings. Furthermore, the arterioles coming off the artery are innervated by free nerve endings that respond to both chemical and mechanical stimulation and can release stored substances that increase vasodilation (Mense 2019).

Taking it from the top

From the fascial tissue at the openings of the nasal passages to the mouth we meet in the pharynx and its attachments to the cranial base.

We continue our descent down a continuous vertical sleeve, along the deepest muscles of the anterior neck (longus colli, longus capitis), until we reach the thorax where it branches out, forming the pleura, which is the fascial skin around the lungs. This also includes a fascial coating around the bronchii inside the lungs (Figure 6.4), which, by the way, if they were removed and flattened, would cover the surface area of a tennis court.

In between the lungs and their pleura is the mediastinum – the connective tissue bag that encloses the heart in front but in the back includes the aorta, esophagus, and trachea. Meanwhile, in the middle of the mediastinum sits the pericardium, which is the epimysium of that most vital muscle, the heart.

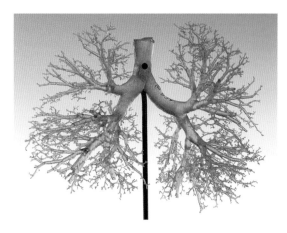

Figure 6.4
The bronchial tree. Casts of lungs, Marco resin, 1951.
Centre for Research Collections University of Edinburgh. Licensed
under the Creative Commons Attribution-Share Alike 2.0 Generic
license: https://creativecommons.org/licenses/by-sa/2.0/deed.en.

The heart as a fascial organ

We learn that the heart is a pump. It is a blood pump that is essential to life. It is a pump where we can track the inflow and outflow of blood to measure its health. Somewhere along the way we forget the heart is a muscle and start treating it like an organ, but the heart is a muscle. That means it has an extracellular matrix (ECM). The predominant components of the cardiac ECM are collagens Type I and III. And excess cardiac collagen has been correlated with myocardial stiffness, as well as diastolic and systolic dysfunctions (Diez et al. 2002).

The muscle tissue of the heart is called myocardia. The most abundant cell in the myocardia is the fibroblast. The cardiac fibroblast performs all the functions one would expect any fibroblast to perform in the fascial net. And when the heart is under extreme duress fibroblasts have been shown to morph via

epithelial-mesenchymal transition (EMT) into cardiac myofibroblasts, which are more mobile, more contractile, and have a greater capacity for producing matrix proteins such as TGF-β1 (Petrov et al. 2002). The possible relationship between ECM remodeling, cardiac fibroblasts, and heart disease is an area of increasing interest (Fan et al. 2012).

Stem-cell-based therapies are also an area of increasing interest. For people whose hearts are too damaged to withstand a heart transplant the only option is usually medication. There is a more experimental option where the patient's own stem cells are injected into the heart to see if that can somehow effect a repair (Mathur & Martin 2004). Oddly, objective tests do not always show measurable improvements in ways that match the positive outcomes some of the test subjects have achieved using stem-cell therapies. Some researchers are concerned, and rightly so, that the data have been misrepresented (Nowbar et al. 2014) and that stem-cell therapy for heart conditions is being hyped for commercial reasons. The systematic review by Nowbar et al. found that trials that showed the most overall positive results also had the largest number of discrepancies. So, for now, this therapy remains controversial.

One surprising area where stem cells have shown positive results is in the regeneration of the heart. Yes, the whole heart. Doris Taylor, currently of the Texas Heart Institute, came up with a "cellular detergent" that removes all the cells but leaves the pericardium intact. This is poetically referred to as the "ghost heart" (Figure 6.5). The first time this was performed was using a rat's heart. Stem cells from the rat were then injected into the matrix and within eight days it was functioning like a regular, healthy heart (Ott et al. 2008).

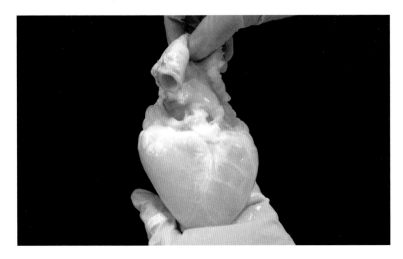

Figure 6.5
The "ghost heart." The pericardium or epimysium, if you prefer, of the heart with all the muscle cells removed. Stem cells have been injected into this fibrillar matrix, and a new heart has been grown.
Image provided by Dr. Doris A. Taylor, Texas Heart Institute, Houston.

Since then, the process has been repeated on both pig and human hearts, with the end goal being able to offer regenerated hearts for transplant, with the organs better able to withstand rejection because they are infused with the cellular stuff of their host. Relatedly, it should be noted that the University of Pittsburgh has been successful at regenerating damaged human muscle by using grafts of animal ECM (Valentin et al. 2010).

Lastly, there is the phenomenon called *increased stroke volume*. Stroke volume is a measurement of how much blood is pumped, per beat, from the left ventricle. Increased stroke volume is sometimes observed with peak athletes during prolonged aerobic activity. During increased stroke volume the blood volume increases but the heart rate goes down. The heart actually enlarges to accommodate the extra blood volume.

This begins to make sense if we alter our view of what the heart really is. German osteopath Gunnar Spohr theorizes that the heart is a "fascial organ." By looking at the heart as a myofascial unit, in this case one without a clear origin or insertion, we move away from a purely mechanical pump model of heart function to a more kinetic, biotensegrity-based model. This further suggests that what we think of as a heartbeat might really be the inherent fascial property of elastic recoil. Such a structure would function more like a spiraling dynament (see Chapter 3) than a pump.

Back to the middle

The tour is not finished yet. The pleura and the mediastinum sit on top of the diaphragm. For the inner fasciae we follow the esophagus down through the hiatus into the abdominal cavity where it splits to form the parietal peritoneum, the fascial lining between the organs, and the body's inner abdominal wall, and then double-bags the rest of the organs. It is worth noting that the mesentery, the double bag of parietal peritoneum that surrounds the small intestine, has now been reclassified as an organ (Coffey & O'Leary 2016).

The parietal peritoneum also serves as a conduit for the nerves, vessels, and lymph. The liver produces between 25 per cent and 50 per cent of all lymph and has an extensive collagen network (Figure 6.6). While providing a skeletal framework, recent evidence suggests the collagen also carves out pathways for fluid flow within the liver (Ohtani & Ohtani 2008).

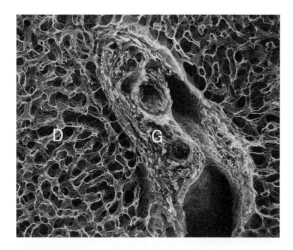

Figure 6.6
The collagen network of the liver, which bears a surprising resemblance to the perimysial and endomysial network in the muscles (see Figure 3.13). Area G is Glisson's capsule – the fascial covering for the portal vein, hepatic artery, and bile duct. Area D shows the individual collagen sheaths for the sinusoid blood vessels of the liver.
Reprinted from Ohtani and Ohtani (2008) with permission from John Wiley & Sons.

Behind all that, or retroperitoneal, are the kidneys. The fascia around the kidneys, referred to as endoabdominal fascia, thickens and forms a fatty pad (also called Gerota's fascia). And for those of you keeping score, the kidneys sit atop the retroperitoneal psoas. Meanwhile, the endoabdominal fascia continues into the endopelvic fascia, which includes the bladder and sexual organs as well as the pelvic diaphragm and "ends" at the levator ani.

The thinking bowel

Since we have looked at the heart as a tensegrity structure, it is only fair to alight upon the bowel as a sensory organ. The network of neural tissue lining the gut is so extensive that some consider it a second brain. There are an estimated 100 million nerve cells in the *enteric* nervous system, lining the alimentary canal from stem to stern. That's more neurons than there are along the spine and in the peripheral nervous system. There are also enteric glia cells (Coelho-Aguiar et al. 2015). Capable of functioning independently of your head brain, the "gut brain" also produces the same array of neurotransmitters as your head brain. Curiously, in Chinese medicine the belly is often referred to as Shen Ch'ue, which means "mind palace." Take that, Sherlock Holmes!

The mind palace was first mapped out by Byron Robinson MD. His book *The Abdominal and Pelvic Brain with Automatic Visceral Ganglia* was first published in 1907 and accurately describes the neurology of a separate brain in the gut. While that volume has faded into obscurity, Robinson's observations were reinforced in Johannis Langley's landmark opus *The Autonomic Nervous System*, first published in 1921.

It was Langley who coined the term "enteric nervous system" and accurately classified the autonomic nervous system into three parts: sympathetic, parasympathetic, and enteric. While the first two classifications are known to every medical student, therapist, and somatic practitioner, the enteric system seemed doomed to obscurity if not for the dogged efforts of Michael Gershon MD to bring prominence to the enteric nervous system in the treatment of digestive disorders.

While it seems most unlikely that we actually reason in a cognitive way with this second brain, the gut brain is so complex that many scientists believe that it could not have possibly developed said complexity solely for moving things down and out through your colon. Philosophically and scientifically, it is being suggested that our gut brain experiences the world in the way our reasoning, cranial brain does not. And in spite of our reliance on reason, the perspective of the gut brain in evaluating reality has equal validity even if it does not involve reason. In the mind–body sense, you cannot reason yourself into being present.

Given the preponderance of gut-related metaphors that have stood the cultural test of time (e.g., a gut feeling, going from the gut, bowels in an uproar, etc.), it should come as no surprise to find these metaphors may have an actual basis in physiological reality. How much our relationship with our enteric nervous system affects our bodies, our cognitive processes, and so on remains to be more fully discovered. As for me, I am of two minds about it.

References

Coelho-Aguiar J de M, Bon-Frauches A C, Gomes A L et al. (2015) The enteric glia: Identity and functions. Glia. June; 63 (6) 921–935.

Coffey J C and O'Leary D P (2016) The mesentery: Structure, function, and role in disease. Lancet Gastroenterol Hepatol. November; 1 (3) 238–247.

Diez J, Querejeta R, López B et al. (2002) Losartan-dependent regression of myocardial fibrosis is associated with reduction of left ventricular chamber stiffness in hypertensive patients. Circulation. May; 105 (21) 2512–2517.

Fan D, Takawale A, Lee J and Kassiri Z (2012) Cardiac fibroblasts, fibrosis and extracellular matrix remodeling in heart disease. Fibrogenesis Tissue Repair. September; 5 (1) 15.

Mathur A and Martin J F (2004) Stem cells and repair of the heart. Lancet. July; 364 (9429) 183–192.

Mense S (2019) Innervation of the thoracolumbar fascia. Eur J Transl Myol. September; 29 (3) 8297.

Nowbar A N, Mielewczik M, Karavassilis M et al. (2014) Discrepancies in autologous bone marrow stem cell trials and enhancement of ejection fraction (DAMASCENE): Weighted regression and meta-analysis. BMJ. April; 348, g2688.

Ohtani O and Ohtani Y (2008) Lymph circulation in the liver. Anat Rec (Hoboken). June; 291 (6) 643–652.

Ott H C, Matthiesen T S, Goh S-K et al. (2008) Perfusion-decellularized matrix: Using nature's platform to engineer a bioartificial heart. Nat Med. January; 14 (2) 213–221.

Petrov V V, Fagard R H and Lijnen P J (2002) Stimulation of collagen production by transforming growth factor-beta1 during differentiation of cardiac fibroblasts to myofibroblasts. Hypertension. February; 39 (2) 258–263.

Stecco L and Stecco C (2013) Fascial Manipulation for Internal Dysfunctions. Padova, Italy: Piccin Nuova Libraria S.p.A.

Valentin J E, Turner N J, Gilbert T W and Badylak S F (2010) Functional skeletal muscle formation with a biologic scaffold. Biomaterials. October; 31 (29) 7475–7484.

Further reading

Barral J-P (1991) The Thorax. Seattle, Washington: Eastland Press.

Barral J-P (2007) Visceral Manipulation II (revised edn). Seattle, WA: Eastland Press.

Barral J-P and Mercier P (2006) Visceral Manipulation (revised edn). Seattle, WA: Eastland Press.

BBC Productions (2010–2011) Horizon: How to mend a broken heart. Documentary.

Chila A (exec. ed.) (2011) Foundations of Osteopathic Medicine. Baltimore & Philadelphia: Lippincott Williams & Wilkins.

Fountain H (2012) Human muscle, regrown on animal scaffolding. The New York Times, September 16, 2012.

Gershon M D (1998) The Second Brain: The Scientific Basis of Gut Instinct and a Groundbreaking New Understanding of Nervous Disorders of the Stomach and Intestine. New York, NY: HarperCollins.

Langley J N (2017) The Autonomic Nervous System, Vol. 1, Classic Reprint Series. London, UK: Forgotten Books.

Marchand P (1951) The anatomy and applied anatomy of the mediastinal fascia. Thorax. December; 6 (4) 359–370.

Robinson B (2017) The Abdominal and Pelvic Brain with Automatic Visceral Ganglia, Classic Reprint Series. London, UK: Forgotten Books.

Shepherd P (2012) New Self, New World: Recovering Our Senses in the Twenty-First Century. Berkeley, CA: North Atlantic Books.

7

Diagnosing Fascial Conditions

If you want to understand function, study structure.

—Francis Crick

Introduction

It was the biannual Fascia Summer School in Leipzig, Germany, and we were under the capable tutelage of the *très magnifique* Danièle-Claude Martin. We were using wooden dowels and rubber bands to build small tensegrity structures. Making tensegrity objects is not hard, but it can be tricky. When one student's structure flew apart for the third or fourth time, Alison Slater (a physiotherapist from Australia) leaned over and said, "I think you've got a tension deficit disorder."

And that could describe most, if not all, fascial problems: TDD – tension deficit disorder.

Fascia responds to mechanical supply and demand, spinning out more collagen for support where needed and secreting enzymes to take collagen away where it is not needed. When excessively mechanically stressed, inflamed, or immobilized (see Figure 1.14), both adhesions and fibrosis can form in the fascia (Langevin 2008). Painful muscle contractions and decreased range of motion are frequently associated with rigid collagenous tissue and other tissues involved in force transmission (Klingler 2012). Dysfunction of the thoracolumbar fascia and tightly contiguous areas, and sometimes not so contiguous, are being recognized as a source of nonspecific low

back pain (Casato et al. 2019). Muscles under chronic concentric contraction will develop denser collagen and often appear "locked short" (Myers 2009). These areas can, and often do, beget other locked-short or locked-long areas that have capacity over time to visibly distort posture as well as create other asymmetries, compensations, and associated tensions.

While anything on the list that follows could have a nonfascial cause, these symptoms tend to be the most common symptoms of fascial dysfunction:

- Decrease in local and/or general range of motion – this tends to involve joints as well as soft tissue around the joint.

- Soft tissue pain when performing simple movements, such as rolling over in bed, putting on a shirt, etc.

- Compromised motor control and lack of co-ordination in simple daily activities, such as walking, tying shoes, etc.

- Reduced flexibility, lack of resilience or "bounce" – just because a joint can be forced to a certain degree in range of motion does not mean that the underlying soft tissue is sufficiently pliable.

- Bad posture or body-wide patterns of compensation and strain.

- Dull aches or pains that never truly go away – the most commonly heard patient complaint by this clinician is: "I do x therapy or y treatment and it feels good for a day, but then it's right back."

- Diminished proprioception and/or interoception – this often manifests as a perceived clumsiness, and the inability to discern subjective or somatic feelings.

So, how do we accurately diagnose or discern dysfunctions with the fascia?

Technology is making this easier, as we shall see, but to begin with let's review methods that have been in use the longest. First, there is postural evaluation or, in more medical parlance, pathoanatomical analysis.

Pathoanatomical analysis

Pathoanatomical analysis (PAA) is a global postural assessment, sometimes casually referred to as "body reading." The essence of PAA is to use the bony landmarks of the body to look for structural asymmetries that appear relevant to the patient's presenting symptoms. More often than not, the relative misalignment of the bony landmarks of the body provides reliably accurate reference points to the areas where the fascia has densified enough to create visible postural distortions. These distortions usually lead to the inability to efficiently use certain muscles and muscle groups, an unbalanced

---

Fascia and cancer

While still quite nascent, there is a growing body of work suggesting a relationship between fascia and cancer (Langevin et al. 2016). Whereas traditional cancer research has focused on halting the neoplastic transformation of cancer cells, recent efforts are starting to focus on the microenvironment of the tumors, and that is where fascia comes in.

First proposed over a century ago (Mueller & Fusenig 2004), and usually referred to in the literature as stroma (the fascial microenvironment), the key element in this relationship is inflammation and tissue stiffness. It seems that these two elements can actually create more neoplastic transformation (Albini & Sporn 2007, Whiteside 2008), increasing tumor growth. So, while body-based, integrative therapies (i.e., massage, yoga, and acupuncture) are being used to improve the symptoms and quality of life of cancer patients, there is also the tantalizing notion that such therapies could potentially serve to assist in ridding the body of cancer.

So far, the evidence is far from conclusive. It has yet to be proven that ECM stiffness by itself can cause tumor proliferation. And tumors have been shown to move both toward and away from areas of higher stiffness (Spill et al. 2016).

Yet there are enough intriguing correlations that in November 2015 the Harvard School of Medicine hosted the first Joint Conference on Acupuncture, Oncology and Fascia. The conference also included explorations of other fascia-oriented manual methods. All the presentations were videoed and are freely available online (Osher Center for Integrative Medicine 2015).

Two things are certain. One is that oncology needs to consider the place of physical medicine in the treatment of cancer. Second, more research is needed on the body-based side to understand the underlying molecular mechanisms so they can be adapted more effectively to the treatment of cancer.

center of gravity, and discernible patterns of strain. Again, these patterns should be easily relatable to the patient and form a plausible hypothesis for why they feel what they feel where they feel it.

Once one learns to observe human structure accurately in this way, it can lead to effective treatment plans that might be missed by working in a symptom-based and/or more regional anatomical mindset. There will be an example of this later in the chapter, but first it is useful to define the terminology.

While I have seen many nomenclatures for describing postural patterns, I am going to borrow the basic terminology of Thomas Myers (2009): It has the virtue of being in simple language and therefore more easily understood by the patient. PAA looks for four specific distortions: shifts, tilts, bends, and rotations.

Shift

A shift is a horizontal displacement of one structure over the other. Figure 7.1 shows a right shift of the rib cage relative to the pelvis, viewed from the frontal plane. Shift also happens in the sagittal view as in Figure 7.2, which illustrates a posterior shift of the rib cage relative to the pelvis.

Tilt

A tilt is a sloping displacement that deviates from the horizontal or vertical. In other words, the body part or bone is higher on one side than the other. Tilts are further delineated by the direction of the slope. Figure 7.3 shows a right tilt of the rib cage, again relative to the pelvis. Figure 7.4 shows an anterior tilt of the pelvis relative to the rib cage, as one might expect to find in a lumbar lordosis.

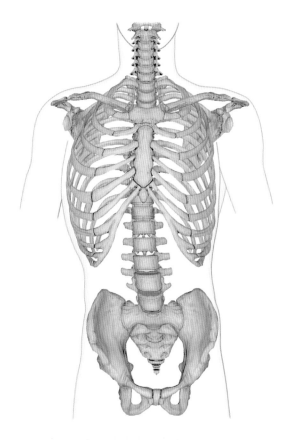

Figure 7.1
A right shift of the rib cage relative to the pelvis underneath. Displacements like this can not only destabilize the shoulder girdle but also change the weight distribution through the legs, further altering force transmission from the foot to the pelvis and beyond.

Bend

A bend is a series of tilts, usually resulting in a curve. One could consider a condition like scoliosis as a series of bends, and overall bends are most commonly seen in the spine. However, lateral bends are also seen in the tibia (Figure 7.5). These presentations suggest a sufficiently densified or

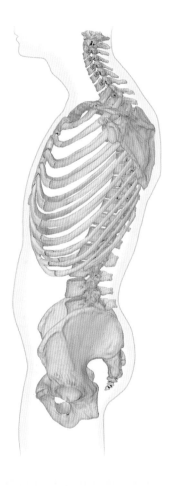

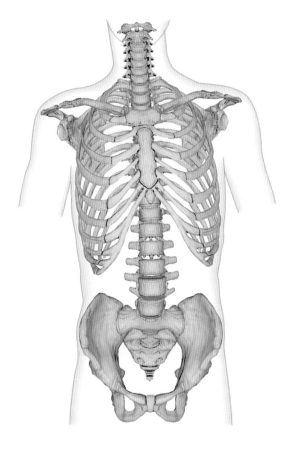

Figure 7.3
A right tilt of the rib cage relative to the pelvis. Pathologies like this are often seen in low back pain and also functional leg length discrepancies.

Figure 7.2
The rib cage posteriorly shifted relative to the pelvis in the sagittal plane. This distortion is often seen in cases of low back pain and is often accompanied by shallow and/or labored breathing in the frontal aspect.

Rotation

A rotation is a displacement that occurs in the transverse, or horizontal, plane. Rotations can often be detected by comparing bony prominences. For example, if one acromion process appears more forward than the other, that could indicate a rotation in the shoulder girdle. The same could be assessed in the hip comparing

restricted deep posterior compartment. Also, a too-tight tibialis anterior can give the appearance of a "banana calf" (Figure 7.6) and often symptomatically manifests as shin splints, knee pain, or just tight calves.

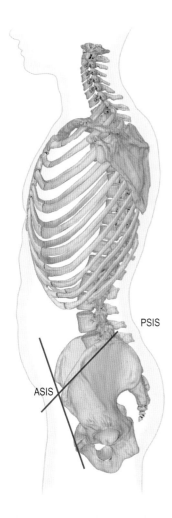

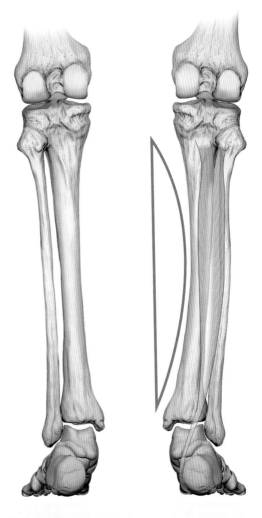

Figure 7.4

An anterior tilt of the pelvis, which can clearly be seen by observing the anterior superior iliac spine "looking" toward the floor. This pattern is again common in low back pain, and also in cases of lumbar spine lordosis, disc compression, and stenosis.

Figure 7.5

Over time, a chronically tightened tibialis posterior can cause the fibula, and to a lesser degree the tibia, to bow out laterally.

the anterior superior iliac spines, and so on throughout the body. An obvious example in our digital age would be an internally rotated humerus and scapula from too much texting or time spent on the computer and would indicate a restricted pectoralis minor (among other culprits).

135

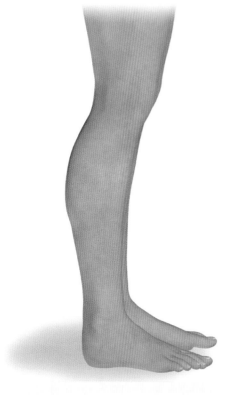

Figure 7.6
The "banana calf," where a chronically shortened tibialis anterior creates a bowing effect, or banana shape, in the reciprocal gastrocnemii and soleus. This pattern often accompanies shin splints, knee strain, and plantar fasciitis.

Deceptively simple, shift, tilt, bend, and rotate when combined can produce body-wide patterns of fascinating complexity and show us where to apply treatment effectively. Usually, these treatment zones will include areas that are less obvious than if the analysis was based solely on the immediate region of symptomatic pain or dysfunction.

Case study: Benjamin

About a year ago, Benjamin began to develop a right-side pain in the area of T8 to T10. In his words, his vertebrae and, in particular, his rib kept "going out." He had been seeing the chiropractor for adjustments. He had also been seeing a physical therapist who was working with him to strengthen his core. While these treatments helped manage his pain, they did not resolve it to his satisfaction. He had been receiving these treatments for a year when he began to seek treatment from me.

The worst activity for Benjamin is sitting, and he is a data-crunching desk jockey. He changed to a kneeling chair at work, and this has helped, but long car trips and plane rides are out of the question for him. Even the idea of a long trip provokes travel anxiety because of the potential for a symptomatic flare-up. Benjamin is 25 years old. I would describe his overall appearance as healthy and fit – but looks can be deceiving.

During the PAA, I was pleased to find his pelvis was perfectly level. A straight line could be drawn from the anterior superior iliac spine to the posterior superior iliac spine in the sagittal plane. His rib cage, however, tilted to the right, drawing it closer to the iliac crest. The rib cage was also rotating to the left, as could be observed by protrusion of the costal margins on the right side. The left costal margins, by comparison, seemed recessed.

From a biotensegrity or fascial perspective this was a tension deficit disorder involving restrictions of the rectus abdominis, aspects of both sets of oblique muscles, the quadratus lumborum, psoas, and diaphragm – all of which served to torque his lower torso in such a way as to cause excessive pull on his ribs at

T8 to T10. This was the pattern underlying Benjamin's pain.

Furthermore, his mid- and lower thoracic spine was showing a slight bend to the right side, following the direction of pull of the abdominal rotation. While the pelvis was level, the bend created a nonsymptomatic strain in the right leg, probably due to an uneven center of gravity. This could be seen in a medial shift of the talus over the calcaneus with a slightly lower medial arch (when compared with the left foot). Also, his gluteals and deeper lateral hip rotators were hypertonic upon palpation.

To reiterate, Benjamin's symptoms were being managed via physical therapy and chiropractic. They were not gone and were still having a significant impact on his quality of life. Any therapeutic treatment plan to achieve a sustained result would have to take all of these forces into consideration.

How could this happen in the first place? We cannot know for certain, but in this case there was another clue in the abdominal region. Underneath his right costal margin was a 2–3 cm long slightly keloidal surgical scar. It turns out Benjamin had had an orthoscopic appendectomy one year prior to the onset of symptoms. He did not mention this initially.

Abdominal adhesions are unavoidable, even in the best orthoscopic surgeries. It is conceivable that Benjamin's pathology began as an adhesion or adhesions from the surgery that altered the force transmission through his torso and was further compounded by the constant compression from his sedentary job. Given that the half-life of collagen is six months, it would take about a year for the symptoms to show up. It is a reasonable hypothesis, although we will

never know for sure. What we do know is that manual treatment of the scar tissue is also now part of his treatment plan due to its efficacy in these types of cases (Bove & Chappelle 2012).

Palpation

Palpation is the art of medical examination through touch, which was first formally recommended by Hippocratic physicians in Ancient Greece as a necessary diagnostic tool. Since then it has fallen in and out of fashion, its fallow periods often predicated by advancements in science and technology that seem to render palpation passé, if not obsolete. Palpation is not obsolete. If anything, it may be missed. I cannot begin to count how many times a new patient will complain to me of doctors and diagnosticians who "never even touched me."

A great deal of useful information can be gathered by palpation, including:

- Muscle tone – weakness or tightness

- Range of motion and "play" in the joint

- Pliability and mobility of the tissue

- Induration, fibrosis, and density of the fascial structures

- Relative differences of those same qualities within the specific muscle, muscle group, or region(s) of the body

- Hot and cold differentials.

Before Tom Findley became an MD and a structural integrator, he fixed and rebuilt car engines. He got so good at it, and his touch became so discriminating, that he could feel an engine valve that was off by 1/32 of an inch. About half a millimeter. And we're capable of even more. Our sense of touch, our ability to use tactile information to process our immediate environment, is the oldest of our senses. Far from that making it the most primitive, its evolutionary age has allowed it to become extraordinarily sensitive and subtle. At the Lipomi Lab at the University of California they wanted to find out just how subtle and sensitive our sense of touch can be (Carpenter et al. 2018).

One factor that can make a difference in our touch is thermal conductivity. How much heat does a given substance draw away from our body? This has an effect on our perception. Let us say we are touching wood or metal. The metal is more conductive and will feel cooler to our touch. Another factor is roughness, so the wood won't feel as smooth as the metal. So, the Lipomi Lab engineered surfaces to counteract those two variables. They further engineered three strips of this surface, except one strip was different. Visually they were identical, but not in thickness. One strip was one molecular layer thicker than the other two. One molecular layer. Test subjects were then asked to identify through touch which one of these things were not like the others. They got it right 71 per cent of the time.

These "sensor readings" from touch come from multimodal mechanoreceptors in the hands and fingers. Each fingertip alone has more than 3,000 touch receptors (Hancock 1995), some of which are quickly responding and paciniform, and others that are slower, low-threshold mechanoreceptors (LTMs) (McGlone et al. 2014). And it's not only the fingertips. Says Darren Lipomi, head of the Lipomi Research Group: "It's not just the mechanoreceptors in the skin but receptors in the ligaments, knuckles, wrist, elbow, and shoulder that could be enabling humans to sense minute differences using touch."

What about sensing touch beyond the fingertips? It turns out that we can do that too.

Just as mice palpate their environment with their whiskers and spiders sense when something tasty is tugging on their webs, we are somehow designed to process sensory information from tools. Be it a hammer, a screwdriver, a butter knife, a gua sha or Graston tool, we are literally wired to feel these objects as extensions of ourselves, of our touch. Tools are sensory extensions of the body (Miller et al. 2018).

Therapeutically it is absolutely vital to combine that sensitive, extensive, inquiring touch with a good working knowledge of anatomy. The better your ability to understand where you are in the body, to visualize the structures under your hands, the more accurate your palpations will be. That combined ability could also be called discriminative touch.

Beyond specific assessments, there is one last tangible benefit that skilled palpation can have on the patient – the benefit of being heard and affirmed. The positive effect of putting one's finger or hand on that exact spot that is hurting and having the patient elicit the "That's it!" response should not be underestimated. The area diagnosed by touch is now real, and not all in their head. And even if some of what is at work here may be the placebo effect, so what if it is?

Therapeutic presence

The concept of "being present" and its many permutations like "mindfulness" (see Chapter 5) or "showing up for your life," etc. ad nauseum is so pervasive these days it is almost a cliché. Back in my day, we called it "paying attention"! Alright, now I'm sounding like the typical grumpy old man. But what if I told you that tactile perception and concentration make a difference to your treatment? It turns out they do.

An ingenious study utilized fMRIs to measure if the attention paid to the quality of touch by the operator/therapist had a demonstrable effect in the person being touched. While both groups touched the same part of the body, one group of operators focused on a series of random auditory beeps delivered via headphones, counting the number of beeps in each delivered sequence. The other group was instructed to focus on the tactile aspects, what they were perceiving from sensory information from their hands. According to the paper these criteria included: consistency, density, temperature, responsiveness, and motility (defined as "myofascial movements"). The results showed that when the toucher sustains their attention on tactile properties it has a significant effect on those being touched (see Chapter 4 for more details). That difference shows up in the areas of the brain involving the processing of interoception (Cerritelli et al. 2017). Not to sound too "woo" but was this the first study to kind of measure intention? It certainly measured attention. More follow-up studies now, please.

Palpation technology

The algometer

A pressure algometer (Figure 7.7) is a low-cost mechanical device for measuring sensitivity to both pressure and pain. Measuring reliably up to 5–6 cm in depth (Park et al. 2011), algometers can easily be used to measure trigger points (Myburgh et al. 2008) both pre- and post-treatment. The measurements have been shown to be quite reliable (Aird et al. 2012).

The MyotonPRO

An expensive, sophisticated device (Figure 7.8), the MyotonPRO utilizes a rapidly pulsating mechanical sensor to record numeric data on

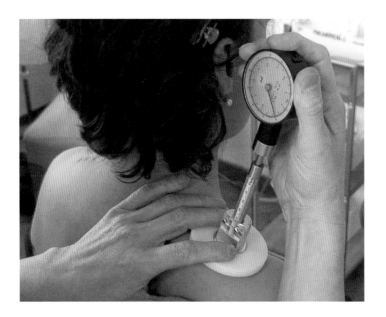

Figure 7.7
Myometry performed with an algometer.
Reproduced with permission from Christopher Gordon.

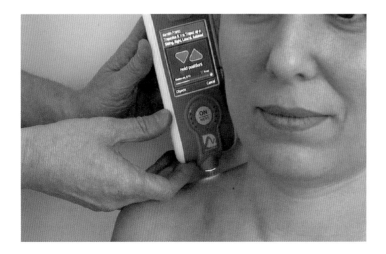

Figure 7.8
Myometry performed with the MyotonPRO.
Reproduced with permission from Christopher Gordon.

tissue properties such as stiffness and elasticity. The measurements have been shown to be quite reliable (Aird et al. 2012). The device itself is quite user-friendly and is sensitive enough to denote deviations in pressure and angle, which virtually eliminates bad data due to operator error.

Imaging technology

Ultrasound

Fascia does not image on X-rays and MRI, but it is observable on ultrasound. Most of us are familiar with ultrasound, which uses high-frequency sound waves to noninvasively penetrate the skin layer so that we can both detect and measure organs and structures inside the body. Ultrasound can visualize and quantify both the superficial and deep fascia, which makes it an excellent diagnostic aide. For example, ultrasound was used to show that the posterior layer, the layer closest to the skin of the thoracolumbar fascia, is on average 25 per cent thicker in those people with low back pain than in healthy people with no LBP (Langevin et al. 2011).

Likewise, another ultrasound study on chronic neck pain found significant differences in the thickness of the fascia of both scalenes and sternocleidomastoid muscles (Stecco et al. 2014). It was further determined that a difference of only 1.5 mm in fascial thickness was a reliable cut-off point to diagnose myofascial neck pain properly.

Ultrasound can show us real-time video of the different fascial layers (Figure 7.9). The same Langevin study (2011) showed a marked difference in "shear strain" – the ability of the different fascial layers to slide relative to each other – in patients with LBP. Watching the different layers sliding or sticking in the case of adhesions while a patient slowly performs lumbar flexion and extension can be quite dramatic. Even more dramatic is being able to take the same ultrasound test after the application of a treatment to that area and being able to both see and measure the improvement in the sliding capabilities of the fascial layers.

Because of these real-time capabilities, some therapists are now using ultrasound to better

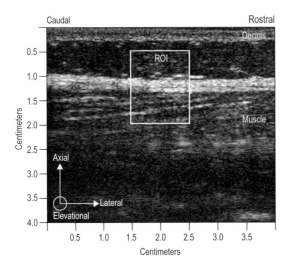

Figure 7.9

Ultrasound elasticity imaging. The white band in the middle of the ROI (region of interest) corresponds with the epimysium. Note the muscle tissue below and superficial fascia above.

From Langevin et al. 2011. Reproduced with permission from BioMed Central.

assess fascial problems and document fascial changes in their patients.

An emerging new development in the field is ultrasound elastography (Drakonaki et al. 2012). Ultrasound elastography has all the advantages of traditional ultrasound but also has the ability to measure tissue stiffness and generate color images (Figure 7.10). The Fascia Research Group at the University of Ulm is using this technology to embark on an ambitious project to determine the normal ranges for fascial stiffness by measuring and analyzing elastographic data taken from large samples of healthy individuals.

At present, both ultrasound and ultrasound elastography equipment is beyond the reach of most clinicians. This is changing as both the technology becomes less expensive and ultrasound manufacturers are becoming more aware of the burgeoning interest from the clinician market. From a research perspective, these advances in measurement technology should lead to greater acceptance of underlying fascial pathologies and also greater efficacy in manual therapy methods.

Oh, and Benjamin is doing much better, too.

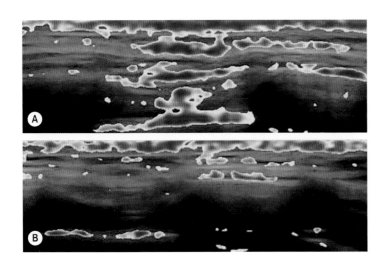

Figure 7.10

Areas of greater tissue stiffness appear as red in ultrasound elastography. The topmost layer, the skin, always exhibits greater stiffness. These two pictures show the same area of the thoracolumbar fascia before (A) and after (B) a therapeutic intervention.

Reproduced with kind permission from Dr. Wolfgang Bauermeister.

References

Aird L, Samuel D and Stokes M (2012) Quadriceps muscle tone, elasticity and stiffness in older males: Reliability and symmetry using the MyotonPRO. Arch Gerontol Geriatr. September–October; 55 (2) e31–e39.

Albini A and Sporn M B (2007) The tumour microenvironment as a target for chemoprevention. Nat Rev Cancer. February; 7 (2) 139–147.

Bove G M and Chapelle S L (2012) Visceral mobilization can lyse and prevent peritoneal adhesions in a rat model. J Bodywork Mov Ther. January; 16 (1) 76–82.

Carpenter C, Dhong C, Root N et al. (2018) Human ability to discriminate surface chemistry by touch. Mater Horiz. 5, 70–77.

Casato G, Stecco C, Busin R (2019) Role of fasciae in nonspecific low back pain. Eur J Transl Myol. August; 29 (3) 159–163.

Cerritelli F, Chiacchiaretta P, Gambi F and Ferretti A (2017) Effect of continuous touch on brain function connectivity is modified by the operator's tactile attention. Front Hum Neurosci. July; 11, 368.

Drakonaki E E, Allen G M and Wilson D J (2012) Ultrasound elastography for musculoskeletal applications. Br J Radiol. November; 85 (1019) 1435–1445.

Hancock E (1995) A handy guide to touch. Johns Hopkins Magazine Electronic Edition. April. Available: http://pages.jh.edu/jhumag/495web/touch.html [May 18, 2022].

Klingler W (2012) Chapter 7.18 Temperature effects on fascia. In: Schleip R, Findley T W, Chaitow L and Huijing P A (eds) Fascia: The Tensional Network of the Human Body. Edinburgh, UK: Churchill Livingstone, Elsevier, pp. 421–424.

Langevin H M (2008) Chapter 6 Potential role of fascia in chronic musculoskeletal pain. In: Audette J F and Bailey A (eds) Integrative Pain Medicine. Totowa, New Jersey: Humana Press, pp. 123–132.

Langevin H M, Fox J R, Koptiuch C et al. (2011) Reduced thoracolumbar shear strain in human chronic low back pain. BMC Musculoskeletal Disorders. September; 12, 203. Available: www.biomedcentral.com/1471-2474/12/203 [May 18, 2022].

Langevin H M, Keely P, Mao J et al. (2016) Connecting (T)issues: How research in fascia biology can impact integrative oncology. Cancer Res. November; 76 (21) 6159–6162.

McGlone F, Wessberg J and Olausson H (2014) Discriminative and affective touch: Sensing and feeling. Neuron. May; 82 (4) 737–755.

Miller L, Montroni L, Koun E et al. (2018) Sensing with tools extends somatosensory processing beyond the body. Nature. September; 561 (7722) 239–242.

Mueller M M and Fusenig N E (2004) Friends or foes – bipolar effects of the tumour stroma in cancer. Nat Rev Cancer. November; 4 (11) 839–849.

Myburgh C, Larsen A H and Hartvigsen J (2008) A systematic critical review of manual palpation for identifying myofascial trigger points: Evidence and clinical significance. Arch Phys Med Rehabil. June; 89 (6) 1169–1176.

Myers T W (2009) Anatomy Trains: Myofascial Meridians for Manual and Movement Therapists, 2nd edn. Edinburgh, UK: Churchill Livingstone Elsevier, p. 21; p. 254.

Osher Center for Integrative Medicine (2015) Joint Conference on Acupuncture, Oncology and Fascia. Video presentations. Available: http://oshercenter.org/joint-conference-2015-video-presentations [May 18, 2022].

Park G, Kim C W, Park S B et al. (2011) Reliability and usefulness of the pressure pain threshold measurement in patients with myofascial pain. Ann Rehabil Med. June; 35 (3) 412–417.

Spill F, Reynolds D S, Kamm R D and Zaman M H (2016) Impact of the physical microenvironment on tumor progression and metastasis. Curr Opin Biotechnol. August; 40, 41–48.

Stecco A, Meneghini A, Stern R et al. (2014) Ultrasonography in myofascial neck pain: Randomized clinical trial for diagnosis and follow-up. Surg Radiol Anat. April; 36 (3) 243–253.

Whiteside T L (2008) The tumor microenvironment and its role in promoting tumor growth. Oncogene. October; 27 (45) 5904–5912.

Further reading

Ingber D E (2008) Can cancer be reversed by engineering the tumor microenvironment? Semin Cancer Biol. October; 18 (5) 356–364.

Schleip R (ed.) (2021) Fascia in Sport and Movement, 2nd edn. Edinburgh, UK: Handspring Publishing, Ch. 20.

Fascia-Oriented Therapies

8

The field of manual therapy is very strongly dominated by the existence of different schools. These schools are usually oriented around very charismatic founders. For example in my school (it was) Ida P. Rolf, the osteopaths around Andrew Taylor Still...these founders had their very profound clinical experiences and they tried to explain them, based on the knowledge of their time, as best as they could.

—Robert Schleip, 2012

There is a popular story attributed to Einstein, which is likely to be apocryphal because I cannot track it down for absolute certain, and it goes something like this. Einstein was giving a lecture or an interview when he was asked: "What do you know for certain?" Einstein paused and said, "Something is moving."

So, what is moving?

For a long time it was believed that fascia-oriented therapies achieved their positive results by simultaneously inducing manual ischemic compression and increasing exothermy until the fascia undergoes a thixotropic phase change and "releases." In simpler terms, the therapist employs pressure and generates heat with their hands until the fascia melts. It feels like that is what is going on, but that is an incorrect interpretation of our palpation. With all we have learned so far it should be obvious that theory cannot be right, and there are even mathematical models (Chaudry et al. 2008) of how much heat and force it would take to cause a plastic tissue deformation of the plantar fascia and the IT band (answer: more than any single human could generate). But those are the two densest fascias in the body. The same study showed that a plastic deformation was possible in the fascia inside the nose, which is

some of the most pliable fascia in the body (think about it), and most of our fascia is somewhere between those extremes.

Often I will be confronted with the question: "So, what are you 'releasing'?" and it's a worthy question. Since release as a term is in the common vernacular among most therapists and many medical professionals it would be difficult to change, but what if we changed what we mean by release? What if we changed the definition? I suggest the following:

A release is the interoceptive, inner sensation of something "letting go" felt by the patient. The interoceptive sensation of release is often accompanied by reduced tension (local or global), overall greater physical ease, improved range of motion, or a combination of these effects. This can also be accompanied by a palpatory change in tissue stiffness on the part of the therapist or practitioner.

This could be caused by responses in the nervous system (autonomic and central, and also proprioceptive and interoceptive), as well as changes to the tissue itself via changes in the gliding properties between layers.

This is yet another example of the "both/and" principle. I am endlessly curious about what is

143

really going on under my hands. What are the mechanisms that generate the positive outcomes that my patients enjoy? When a positive outcome does not happen, what is changing or blocking those processes? How can new knowledge modify our approach?

Put a crimp in your style

Something we do understand to be important is the two-directional, latticed architectural aspect of fascia. Think of the warp and weft in nylon hosiery, which gives it both stretch and strength. The more regular the lattice, the better the crimp of the individual collagen fibers. Crimp is the wavy springiness of the individual collagen fibers that allow for their proper flexion–extension along the stress–strain curve (see Chapter 2). Healthy two-directional lattice formation accounts for the greater springiness and elasticity found in the movement of young people (Staubesand et al. 1997). Losing that spring in our step as we get older and more sedentary causes the crimp to become disorganized and random (Figure 8.1).

Studies with animals (Järvinen et al. 2002) show that immobility promotes crosslinks in the fascial tissues, essentially making them stuck and matted together. Tissues in this state lose their ability to glide. It is thought that the proper stimulation of the fibroblasts through movement can promote restoration of healthy crimp and glide (Müller & Schleip 2012). I would also speculate the same is true in our manual therapies.

Macro to micro: Fascial release at the cellular level

While the preceding chapters have explored many of the mechanisms at play in the fascial web and how they function, one of the most

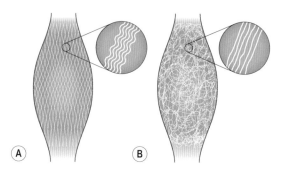

Figure 8.1

Collagen architecture responds to loading. Fasciae of young people (A) express more often a clear two-directional (lattice) orientation of their collagen fiber network. In addition, the individual collagen fibers show a stronger crimp formation. As evidenced by animal studies, application of proper exercise can induce an altered architecture with increased crimp formation. Lack of exercise on the other hand, has been shown to induce a multidirectional fiber network and a decreased crimp formation (B).

Illustration adapted with permission from fascialnet.com.

intriguing experiments attempting to model myofascial release (MFR) was carried out on the cellular level (Meltzer et al. 2010). The monofilaments, intermediate filaments, and microtubules that make up the cytoskeleton are mechanically active and will respond to stress. In Melzer's simulation, active cell cultures of human fibroblasts were subjected to eight hours of repetitive motion strain (RMS) using a vacuum-driven, flexible petri dish apparatus. That same apparatus was then reconfigured to approximate MFR by simulating compression (load) with strain (uniaxial stretch) over a sustained period of 60 seconds (time).

The fibroblasts subjected to RMS exhibited elongated lamellipodia, cellular decentralization, cytoplasmic condensation, and reduced cell-to-cell contact area. Most significant was a 30 per cent increase in fibroblast apoptosis (cell death) among the RMS group when compared with the nonstressed control and other groups (Figure 8.2).

The RMS fibroblasts that received 60 seconds of MFR not only reduced apoptosis to slightly below the level of the nonstressed control group, but also mostly restored the other negative factors to near their prestressed levels.

Clearly something is moving.

Fascia modalities

What follows are the basics for a wide range of fascia-related modalities, presented in a user-friendly way. While it is generally accepted that

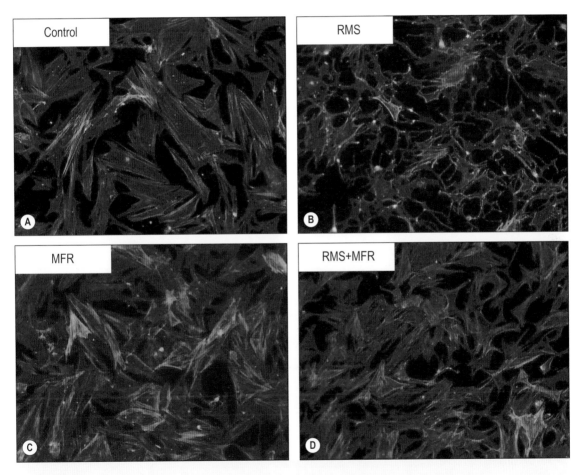

Figure 8.2
Results of the experiment attempting to model myofascial release at the cellular level. (A) The control group shows healthy fibroblast and actin architecture. (B) RMS is the repetitive motion strain group. (C) MFR is the healthy group that received myofascial release. (D) The image shows a culture that had induced RMS and then MFR.
Reprinted from Meltzer et al. (2010) with permission from Elsevier.

all of these treatments can positively affect the fascia, inclusion is neither meant as endorsement nor that the therapy has been conclusively proven to work through evidence-based or randomized clinical trials. To quote Leon Chaitow: "Lack of proof of efficacy is not the same as proof of lack of efficacy." They are included because they have a reputation for getting the desired results.

Acupuncture

Origin: According to archaeological evidence, acupuncture dates back to the Neolithic Age, somewhere between 10,000 and 2,000 BCE, and the original needles were made of stone (Deng & Cheng 1996). From there, and to suit our purpose, we need to time-travel considerably into the future to 2001 and the laboratory of Helene Langevin. Professor Langevin has long been intrigued by the "grasping" sensation often associated with acupuncture. This is the physiologic sensation felt by the fingers of the practitioner of the acupuncture needle being sucked into the body by the tissue. It has no biological explanation, or at least none until very recently (Langevin et al. 2001).

What was observed under the microscope was loose connective tissue wrapping itself around the acupuncture needle. Every time the needle was twisted, the loose connective tissue would further entwine itself, like "spaghetti around a fork" (Figure 8.3) (Langevin et al. 2002). Furthermore, this phenomenon also occurs in living tissue (Langevin et al. 2004). It is precisely this kind of stretch that activates mechanotransduction and has an effect on the shape of nearby fibroblasts (Langevin et al. 2011).

Methods: In acupuncture, very fine needles, about the width of a human hair, are inserted into the skin. The insertion is not at random: the acupuncture points occur along 20 specific

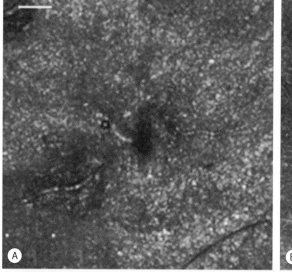
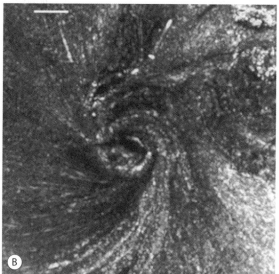

Figure 8.3
Ultrasound scan of subcutaneous tissue during acupuncture. The "black hole" is the area of needle insertion. (A) The area with no rotation; (B) shows the same area when under unidirectional needle rotation.
Reprinted from Langevin et al. (2002) with permission from John Wiley & Sons.

lines throughout the body called meridians. These meridians are the conveyors of qi, often spelled, and pronounced, "chi." In traditional Chinese medicine, qi is the essential energy of the human body. Qi maintains all the vital and functional activities of tissues and organs.

The meridians themselves seem to have a deeper connection to the fascia, as they appear to be preferentially located along fascial planes. More than 80 per cent of the acupuncture points in the arm are located along fascial planes (Langevin & Yandow 2002). The meridians also a display close relationships to the myofascial meridians (see Chapter 3 and also Myers 2020).

In practice: Acupuncture treatment is usually goal-oriented, centered around achieving sustained results for a wide variety of autoimmune, systemic, and musculoskeletal pains. It has been shown to be quite effective for chemotherapy-related vomiting and idiopathic headaches (Ernst 2009). The pulse at the wrist is felt for various qualities that indicate excesses and deficiencies in the meridians. A visual examination of the tongue is also quite common. This information will be correlated with presenting symptoms to determine which meridians and acupuncture points will be stimulated.

Upon insertion, the patient may not even feel the needles; they may elicit the briefest of jabs, but that sensation passes within seconds. Many people report warm or heavy sensations at the insertion point. The needles are then left in for a period of anywhere from 15 to 60 minutes. The number of treatments required to achieve a sustained result varies with the condition.

Learn more: International Academy of Medical Acupuncture, Inc. At: https://iama.edu

Bowen technique

Origins: Tom Bowen created this form of bodywork in Geelong, Victoria, Australia. Born in Australia of British parents, Tom worked at the local cement plant and had no formal training of any kind. It should also be noted that he was profoundly deaf. There does not appear to be any record of how he discovered his ability or refined his process. He regarded it as "a gift from God." There are accounts of Tom treating dozens of people in his home during the evening hours, traveling to sports clubs all over Geelong to treat footballers on the weekends, and making his services available to the local police, so much so that they made him an honorary member of the Geelong Crime Car Squad. He would pass down his knowledge to six individuals who would continue working in his method, two of whom would open a free children's clinic. Tom died in 1982.

Methods: Bowen has a series of "moves" almost always beginning with a gentle lumbar decompression to facilitate a change to a more parasympathetic state. The moves are often applied to the musculotendinous junctions, where the muscle tendon meets the bone, and are performed in a specific sequence of finding where the slack is in the area, applying gentle pressure, and rolling the area in tension toward greater ease. These moves are usually stacked together in small groups of no more than four to six moves. Then, a five-minute break or "therapeutic pause" occurs to allow the person being treated, and their nervous system, time to process and respond. Typically, unless otherwise requested, the Bowen practitioner leaves the room during this time. Upon returning, another series of moves is employed, usually based on how the body has responded to the previous set. From a fascia perspective, it is theorized that one of the mechanisms involves stimulating the sensory nerves that are so abundant in the superficial fascia. It is further theorized that the break between moves allows greater time for interoception.

In practice: Bowen is well known for the overall gentleness of its therapeutic approach. The person undergoing treatment should arrive in loose, comfortable clothing as they stay clothed for the duration of the session. Ten sessions five to ten days apart are usually recommended for the best overall results. While Bowen has not been widely studied, a randomized controlled trial conducted on 120 asymptomatic nonprofessional athletes showed a measurable change in hamstring flexibility both post-treatment and up to one week later (Marr et al. 2011).

Learn more: www.bowen-academy.com or www.bowencollege.com

Fascial Fitness®

Origins: Fascial Fitness® (FF) began as a collaboration between continuum movement teacher Divo Müller and Robert Schleip as a way to directly apply the research on fascia to the world of sports and exercise (Schleip & Müller 2013). For example, correlations between the high kinetic storage capacity of kangaroo tendons as the reason for their high jumping abilities (Kram & Dawson 1988) and ultrasound examinations showing a similar elastic catapult capacity in the human Achilles tendon and associated aponeuroses (Sawicki et al. 2009). The goal of FF is to increase resilience throughout the entire fascial net and minimize injuries.

Methods: FF has four key components. These are elastic recoil, fascial stretch, fascial release, and proprioceptive refinement.

Elastic recoil: Elastic recoil requires an adequate preparatory countermovement. Like a bowstring needing the right amount of tension in order for the arrow to meet its mark, the preparatory countermovement tenses the fascia in the opposite direction of the desired movement for a springier, more energy-efficient movement. These exercises often employ kettle bells, weights, and rhythmic bouncing.

Fascial stretch: Fascial stretch involves engaging in flowing, rather than static, full-body stretches that engage long myofascial chains. In many ways these stretches are similar to what animals do instinctively, and those of you with pets will see this all the time. Stretches of this nature are known as pandiculations (Bertolucci 2011).

Fascial release: Using rollers of different viscosity and very slow movement, fascial release is utilized to relax and rehydrate fascial tissues. Conversely, more rapid rolling could be utilized before an athletic endeavor to stimulate proprioception and improve performance.

Proprioceptive refinement: This is induced by both slow and fast micromovements. Sometimes these are lightly loaded. Key to this component is an exploratory mindset and focusing attention on the quality of movement.

In practice: FF classes are structured like any good exercise class, proceeding from warm-up to maximum effort, followed by gentle cooldown. Because of stimulating the fascia in this manner and the cycle of collagen turnover (Kjaer et al. 2009, Magnusson et al. 2010), too much fascial training could have the exact opposite effect, so it is recommended that this kind of training be done only twice a week. Furthermore, once the principles of FF are sufficiently understood, they may be applied to any exercise routine or sports endeavor.

Learn more: https://fasciatrainingacademy.com/fascial-fitness-training

Fascial Manipulation®

Origins: Fascial Manipulation® (FM) was developed by Italian physiotherapist Luigi Stecco. It takes into account the role of fascia in motor control and also the control of posture. Luigi's children, Carla and Antonio, have followed in their father's footsteps by going into the family business. They have both furthered the field of fascia science by virtue of their meticulous research into the histology, innervation, and anatomy of fascia.

Methods: FM divides the body into 14 functional segments (Figure 8.4). Each functional segment is governed by six myofascial units (MFUs). MFUs are functional units responsible for controlling the movement of that segment. MFUs comprise:

- Motor units innervating mono- and biarticular muscle fibers

- A joint that moves unilaterally when those fibers contract

- Fascia that connect the fibers to ligament, tendon, joint capsules, and menisci

- Nerves involved in the contraction.

Each MFU is further divided into two different areas. The first is called the center of coordination (CC) and is the active component of the MFU. The CC is located in a small area in the deep fascia of the muscle belly where muscle fiber contraction takes place.

The passive element of the MFU is called the center of perception (CP). The CP is where traction from the contractile fibers is perceived and

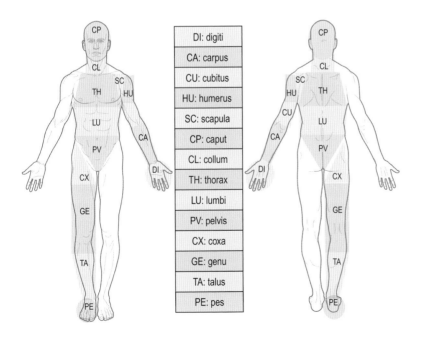

| DI: digiti |
| CA: carpus |
| CU: cubitus |
| HU: humerus |
| SC: scapula |
| CP: caput |
| CL: collum |
| TH: thorax |
| LU: lumbi |
| PV: pelvis |
| CX: coxa |
| GE: genu |
| TA: talus |
| PE: pes |

Figure 8.4

The 14 functional segments used in Fascial Manipulation® with their associated Latin names and abbreviations.

Reproduced from Chaitow (2014) with permission from Handspring Publishing.

is found in the joint capsule, ligament, or tendon. The CP almost always correlates to where the patient is describing symptoms.

This method also has unique nomenclature for describing natural movement. This was created to streamline and simplify the terminology for both patient and practitioner.

In practice: Assessment involves taking a symptomatic history with detailed chronology to best understand the sequelae of injury and compensation leading to the presenting symptom(s). Then, both movement and palpation assessments are utilized to determine which functional segments and CCs are involved in the pathology.

Treatment consists of deep crossfiber friction applied to the densified CCs. The goal is to restore elasticity and proper sliding (via local increase of hyaluronan). The immediate goal is to relieve the pain, with the longer-term aim being to resolve the dysfunction in as few treatments as possible.

Learn more: www.fascialmanipulation.com

Frederick Stretch Therapy™

Origins: Frederick Stretch Therapy™ (FST) is the cocreation of Ann and Chris Frederick. Ann credits her education in kinesiology to having grown up in her mother's dance studio from the age of four. A professional dancer and dance teacher, Ann started developing FST in 1995 at Arizona State University. In 1996 she created FST for the US men's Olympic wrestling team.

Coming from the world of physical therapy, and a professional ballet dancer in his own right, Chris began studying FST with Ann in 1998, and he liked it so much that he married her! Together they evolved FST into the sophisticated neuro-myofascial manual therapy and movement re-education system that it is today.

Methods: The basis for FST involves stretch with sustained traction of the joint capsule and myofascia combined with slow oscillations and circumductions in multiple planes of movement. Often the lower limb is comfortably secured under a series of soft straps to better increase leverage and more accurately target the specific joint or neuromyofascial unit. "No pain, no pain" is a mantra of FST, as the positive gains need to be made by finesse not by force.

One of the other keys to the method is the metaphor of the stretch wave. The stretch wave concept is to help practitioners and patients to understand stretch as a series of undulations of movement coordinated with proper breathing. Proper breathing is essential in the FST model for both practitioner and patient.

In practice: Assessment begins with the usual medical history followed by a number of objective tests involving both dynamic and static palpation. Other measures include, but are not limited to, posture, gait, observation of activities of daily living, and other movement patterns. In a nutshell, the FST practitioner is looking for what can be shortened or lengthened or stabilized to achieve the goals of the session. FST sessions can last anywhere from 15 to 120 minutes. FST is used both to resolve longstanding pain and functional issues as well as specific protocols for enhancing the performance of professional athletes. FST adjusts the parameters to fit the needs of the client and can be used in rehabilitation and recovery to correct imbalances or to prepare for imminent athletic activity.

Learn more: http://stretchtowin.com

John F. Barnes' Myofascial Release Approach®

Origins: John Barnes was working as a young physical therapist when via a weightlifting accident he crushed several discs in his lumbar spine. He underwent lumbar fusion surgery to remedy the situation with subsequent physical therapy to address the problem, but the therapy did not work – at least not fully. John still came home from work in pain every day.

The only thing that would give him relief was lying on the floor and using his own body weight and leverage to apply pressure to the affected areas. He found that maintaining sustained pressure over a period of several minutes would relieve the pain, and with repeat applications the pain continued to be relieved for longer and longer cumulative durations. As he began to see the benefits in himself, he began to create manual methods to apply these same compressive principles to his physical therapy patients.

Methods: The Barnes Approach has three distinct facets: structural, unwinding, and rebounding.

Structural: The structural part of the approach involves the more compressive, hands-on techniques applied to areas of fascial restrictions. Therapists take up the slack of the muscular component, then feel for the collagenous barrier (densification). They then apply steady continuous pressure at that level for at least three to five minutes, and often longer, to facilitate a thorough release via increasing both depth into the body and elongation of the tissue.

Unwinding: Unwinding, or myofascial movement facilitation, involves fully supporting a limb or area of the body in order to nullify the effects of gravity upon it. This often returns the body to the original position and/or tensile state experienced during the trauma. Unwinding often happens spontaneously. The therapist follows the inherent movement along the path of least resistance until it stops. This is called the still point, as all physiologic motion ceases. Often at the still point there can be accompanying somatoemotional release.

Rebounding: Myofascial rebounding involves working with the fluid dynamics and elastic recoil properties of fascia to induce an oscillation through the fascial net that helps to reset the nervous system component through distraction and confusion. In this respect it could be said to be somewhat analogous to eye movement desensitization and reprocessing (EMDR) therapy, which is used to treat aspects of post-traumatic stress disorder (PTSD) (Servan-Schreiber 2005) by changing the way the nervous system processes stressful information.

In practice: This approach always starts with an array of assessments: postural, range of motion, gait, etc. A treatment plan is then devised that involves two sessions of 30–60 minutes per week. Regular reassessments occur throughout the sessions. Every third treatment has a strong self-care focus, using balls, rollers, and long pandiculating stretches (to simulate unwinding), so that the patient can become better empowered, with the ultimate goal being independence from the therapist.

Learn more: https://myofascialrelease.com

Foam Rolling aka Self-Myofascial Release (SMFR)

Origins: While no one can say for sure, or at least I can't, when the first foam roller appeared, there is no doubt that we humans have been using inanimate objects to help ease out aches and pains for a long time. In science we call these objects stress transfer mediums (STMs). But these tools, be they balls, rollers, or something else altogether, give us the real-time opportunity to explore our proprioception as well. Benefits of SMFR supported by current research include improved range of motion, improved neuromuscular coordination, decrease of both muscle fatigue and delayed onset muscle soreness (DOMS), improved vascular function, and an increase in the parasympathetic response (Miller 2021).

Methods: SMFR uses both soft foam rollers and a variety of balls of different sizes and viscosities to mimic the techniques and results of hands-on manual therapies. Different densities may be better for different areas of the body, and this will likely vary from individual to individual. One important factor is tool hardness, with newer studies indicating that softer is better (Kim et al. 2019). Too firm and you can actually damage your tissue. Likewise, there is no consensus on how much pressure is appropriate, but it is recommended to avoid the guideline to use "maximum tolerable pressure." Use the amount of pressure that feels productive or necessary. To simplify – if you are wincing you are doing it wrong. It does not have to hurt to work.

In practice: Go slow, please, and be reasonable. I once had a patient come to me diagnosed with IT band syndrome that wasn't getting any better. A highly motivated individual, who once trained to climb Mount Kilimanjaro, he did not understand why his condition had not improved when he had been doing SMFR on his IT band every day for 30 minutes for a period of one month. There is such a thing as overdoing it. This author recommends that you get some guidance, take a class or two (in person or online), and develop

a better understanding of how you can get the most out of SMFR. Some of the more thorough methods include, but are not limited to, MELT Method, Tune-Up Fitness, and Yamuna.

Learn more: see Further reading

Merrithew™ Fascial Movement

Origins: PJ O'Clair has been involved in the fitness industry since the mid-1980s. She got her first appreciation for fascia in the early 2000s, working in the dissection labs at Tufts Medical, Boston, with Gil Headley and Todd Garcia. Intrigued by the sliding and gliding layers under her hands and scalpel, she began to conceive of the idea of creating a movement class to accentuate that fascial aspect of the body. Already a well-respected Pilates and yoga teacher, PJ knew she would need to incorporate aspects of both of those systems into the new technique, and that it would not look like either of them. She also knew that music with mindful movement would play a role.

This led her to collaborate with multiple Latin Grammy-winning composer Kike Santander. Santander's vision was to bring his Zen-like music to the fitness industry with choreographed sequences written by PJ and her programming team. This collaboration evolved into the Mindful Movement program known as ZEN·GA®.

Merrithew™ Fascial Movement (MFM) is the next evolution. Whereas ZEN·GA® focuses more on softer, more relaxing qualities of fascial-based protocols, MFM combines the latest research to create more resilience, as well as awareness, in the fascial body. MFM can strengthen and tone the fascia as well as restore it.

Methods: The basis for MFM involves four fascia movement variables: bounce, sense, expand, and hydrate.

Bounce: Bounce seeks to develop spring-like, effortless actions in rhythmic movements. Pre-tension, recoil, and the stretch-shortening cycle are all used to foster this capability within the fascia, from superficial to the deepest visceral layer. Music, of course, plays a key role. There are both strengthening and restorative applications.

Sense: Using props and tools with various textures, vibrations, and FlexBands of differing viscoelasticity, sense has a more neurological component and stimulates both proprioception and interoception. Breathing awareness also plays a key role.

Expand: Expand actively explores force transmission and promotes better tissue glide and fluid flow. Breathing awareness again has a key role, particularly using hydraulic expansion to activate better core stability. Pandiculations (whole body stretches) are used throughout.

Hydrate: Hydrate assists optimal force transmission by enhancing glide and hydration for greater ease in movement. Hydrate uses soft and firm rollers and balls to "soak and squeeze" the fascial tissues. Hydrate seeks also to promote capillary flow, thereby improving arterial flow and venous return.

In practice: MFM is taught both in groups and one-on-one. From an instructor standpoint, MFM training allows for specific classes with myriad programming options. Once the core concepts of MFM are understood, they can be easily integrated into any movement, fitness, or sports endeavor at any level.

Learn more: https://merrithew.com

Myofascial Trigger Point Therapy

Origins: Myofascial Trigger Point Therapy was developed by Dr. Janet Travell. As a young doctor she found that many of her patients with pulmonary disease complained of terrible shoulder and arm pain. Methodical palpation of the chest, arms, and shoulders revealed to Dr. Travell the presence of trigger zones (Travell 1968). She would trace these painful areas to trigger points – hyperirritable nodules located within a taut band of skeletal muscle (Travell & Simons 1999a), colloquially referred to as muscle knots.

Dr. Travell would soon abandon cardiology to focus on the etiology of these muscle knots. Partnering with Dr. David Simons, the two of them produced a thorough topographic documentation of trigger points and their patterns of referred pain (pain felt in areas adjacent to the trigger point). This information can be found in their two-volume, 2,000-plus-page treatise *Myofascial Pain and Dysfunction* (Travell & Simons 1999a, 1999b).

Trigger points can be latent; that is, someone can have them and not experience pain (rather like the segment of the population with disc issues but no pain). It has been shown that biochemicals associated with pain, inflammation, and intercellular signaling are present near active trigger points (Shah & Gilliams 2008).

Methods: The basic method for Myofascial Trigger Point Therapy is ischemic compression performed by the finger(s), hand, arm, or even elbow of the therapist. Pressure is applied to the point where initial resistance is felt and then sustained until the trigger point begins to soften. This melting sensation is often felt both by the patient and the therapist. Trigger points may also be treated in a manner similar to acupuncture with a therapy called dry needling.

In practice: While many trigger point therapists often use other adjunct therapies, they typically have excellent palpation skills. This is a must for finding the exact location of the taut bands and tender nodules and also for being able to provide just the right amount of pressure to elicit the desired effect without causing more pain in the process. Various stretch-based protocols are also part of the rehab process.

Learn more: National Association of Myofascial Trigger Point Therapists. At: www.myofascialtherapy.org

Structural Integration

Origins: Structural Integration (SI) was created by Ida Rolf. When Ida was a child, she contracted pneumonia and a raging fever after a nearly fatal kick from a horse. Her health and vitality were restored after having her spine manipulated by an osteopath from Montana (Love 2011). Ida graduated from Columbia University with a PhD in organic chemistry in 1921 – just one year after women in the USA were given the right to vote. She went on to become the first woman to hold a research post at the Rockefeller Foundation (Jacobson 2011).

Ida discovered hatha yoga at the Clarkstown Country Club in Nyack, New York, and would remain a lifelong devotee. She studied homeopathy in Europe and was also strongly influenced by somatic pioneer Alfred Korzybski as well as a number of osteopaths, including William Sutherland. In the 1950s she would begin teaching her first hands-on classes in structural dynamics at the European College of Osteopathy in Maidstone, England. As she developed her hands-on approach, she would name this process "Structural Integration."

Methods: The SI process centers on reorganizing the human being in the field of gravity to achieve better balance, proper alignment, and ease of motion. Given recent inquiries into the ability of the cytoskeleton, the structural component of the cell, to sense gravity and mechanotransduction itself as a cellular adaptation to gravity, this notion may not be as far out as it once seemed (Vorselen et al. 2014, Najrana & Sanchez-Esteban 2016). Fundamental to this process is recognizing fascia as the primary organ of structure. Static postural examinations are routine.

SI is based on a repeatable sequence known as "the recipe" – a series of ten sessions designed by Ida Rolf that have specific physiological goals. The exact sequence of each session is modified by virtue of the individual, idiosyncratic asymmetries of the patient. The overarching goal of the ten sessions is to achieve a balanced tone, or palintonicity, throughout the biotensegrity of the body. Rolf would also develop a movement-based practice to complement SI in collaboration with Dorothy Nolte and Judith Aston.

The fascial changes are produced by slow, hands-on fascial and myofascial releases that also involve slow stretches and guided movements on the part of the patient.

In practice: Actual mileage varies. Some practitioners treat SI as a step-by-step realignment and fundamental movement re-education process for the human body. Others use the basic recipe as a jumping-off point to treat a variety of chronic pain and musculoskeletal disorders.

Different schools have different approaches. For example, Hellerwork® has a paradigm that is designed to address the psychoemotional, as well as biomechanical, aspects of the patient and has an 11th session. Anatomy Trains Structural Integration (ATSI®) has 12 sessions, and takes an anatomically rigorous approach via the Anatomy Trains model of force transmission.

It should also be noted that "Structural Integration" is a generic term. Names such as Rolfing®, Hellerwork®, or ATSI® denote a particular brand of SI-influenced therapy. While the fundamentals are similar, the individual expressions can be different.

Learn more: International Association of Structural Integrators®. At: www.theiasi.net

Visceral Manipulation

Origins: Visceral Manipulation (VM) was developed by French osteopath and physical therapist Jean-Pierre Barral. While working as a young physician, Barral found that he could relieve certain aches and pains simply by kneading the organs (Barral 2008). At that time, practitioners of osteopathy were not interested in manipulating the organs so much as manipulating the spine, so for Barral it was wide-open territory.

His attention to thoroughly documenting his methods and their results resulted in a gradual consistency in treating conditions like chronic indigestion, incontinence, migraines, reflux, IBS, and more. The techniques Barral pioneered and refined are now part of the standard curriculum at all osteopathic colleges in Europe.

Methods: The basis for VM is that the natural, inherent physiologic motion of the organs is basic to their healthy functioning.

Visceral mobility: Visceral mobility refers to the motion of the viscera in response to voluntary movements: walking, running, bending over, the up-and-down motion of the diaphragm during respiration, and so on. If the ligaments of the organs are compromised or the organs are not sliding in the serous membranes (as can happen with scar tissue after abdominal surgeries) function will be compromised. Visceral restrictions can also manifest as neuromuscular pain, as in the case of chronic right-side-only shoulder pain having a relationship to the falciform ligament of the liver (Barral 1991).

Visceral motility: Visceral motility refers to the intrinsic, active motion of the organs. The movement cycle has two phases: toward and away from the midline of the body. Motility is a slow, low amplitude movement that is assessed solely through very sensitive palpation. Barral admits to motility having no scientific explanation, but he is aware of it from palpatory observations over four decades of clinical experience. He speculates that it may have a relationship with the craniosacral rhythm.

VM is performed with the hands using soft pressure. Often, slow, guided stretching is part of the technique.

In practice: VM sessions are usually very gentle, as befits the delicacy of the tissues involved. They are usually 45–60 minutes in duration and spaced several weeks apart. Highly chronic situations may involve greater frequency, and sometimes teaching the patient self-care may be warranted.

Learn more: www.barralinstitute.com

Yin yoga

Origins: The introduction of yin yoga to the West happened in the late 1970s and is credited to yogi and martial artist, Paulie Zink. It has its roots in Taoist yoga, which Paulie was an adherent of, where the asanas (yoga poses) are held for longer periods of time than traditional hatha styles of yoga. This form of yoga has been further popularized in the US by Paul Grilley and Sarah Powers. Paul has infused the style with a stronger anatomical foundation. Sarah has brought to it more traditional Chinese medicine concepts, including more dynamic sequences and postures designed to enhance the flow of qi through the meridians.

Methods: While most forms of yoga do work the fascia (how can they not?), they tend to be more energetic and thus considered yang. However, yin yoga has a slower, more contemplative pace. The slower pace is thought to foster an inner stillness, among other spiritual goals. While the asanas are similar to other forms of yoga, they often have different names and are modified to engender a relaxation, as opposed to exertion, effect in the muscles. It is this quality along with the duration of the poses that is thought to produce a beneficial effect on the connective tissue and also serves to rehydrate the fascia.

In practice: Yin yoga classes function much like any other yoga class; however, the asanas are typically held for three to five minutes, and occasionally longer, depending on the pose. As such, there are fewer poses in a yin class than in more hatha-oriented styles of yoga. The goal is to passively create length and flexibility.

Learn more: see Further reading

General guidelines for exercise and diet

Collagen supplements

At the time of this writing the branding of collagen supplements is at an all-time high. Not to mention bone broth. Hasn't broth always been bone-based? Anyway, what can we really say about the efficacy of collagen supplementation at this time? The preliminary data is quite promising.

Marketing around collagen supplements has traditionally been hyped as making our skin look better as we age. In the more therapeutic realm, a 2018 review on supplements specific to improving adaptation and recovery in athletes (Rawson et al. 2018) looked at four studies and cautiously concluded that there "could" be a benefit in supplementation that focused on connective tissue. A more robust literature review looking at over 60 studies (Juher & Pérez 2015) concluded that hydrolyzed collagen supplementation increases collagen synthesis as well as glycosaminoglycans and hyaluronan, although there is also the point of view that a healthy diet rich in proteins and amino acids should obviate the need for additional supplementation. But how does your body "know" where to direct the collagen it ingests? Mechanotransduction and one other element seem to be crucial.

Professor Keith Baar at the University of California, Davis School of Medicine has developed a formula that works well for rehabilitating injured athletes (Steffen & Baar 2021). I recommend it to patients who have all sorts of musculoskeletal injuries. It is very specific:

- Hydrolyzed collagen (HC) only – 0.2 grams HC for every kilogram of weight

- 50 mg of vitamin C, which is necessary for catalyzation. (Keith suggests dissolving the HC in a glass of orange juice.)

- Load tissue within 45 minutes of ingestion.

So do the math, drink it and go for a walk. Or go to the gym, or do yoga – whatever loading strikes your fancy. This can be repeated throughout the day with no adverse effects.

The Mayo Clinic lists only three possible side effects from collagen supplementation:

1. Possible allergic reaction from marine-derived collagen (if you have a shellfish allergy).

2. Possible bad aftertaste in the mouth.

3. Higher than normal calcium levels, leading to constipation.

That last one ought to be easy enough to self-monitor.

Exercise and fitness

It is becoming more accepted that exercise that includes a facial component is important for building better health and resiliency. In general, any form of fitness that emphasizes full body pandiculation-oriented movements are recommended. This quality, along with the attention paid to the quality of how and what our body feels when moving, make both yoga and Pilates ideal.

Adding fascia-focused elements (elastic recoil, bounce, etc.) as outlined in the previous sections on fascial fitness and fascial movement to the current regimen can also result in positive gains. To give more specific directions would require another book. Fortunately, that book exists, the second edition of *Fascia in Sport and Movement* (see Further reading: Schleip & Wilke 2021). With over two dozen specific sport and fitness focused chapters, plus many others on fascial foundations, you will discover many, many key insights.

References

Barral J-P (1991) The Thorax. Seattle, WA: Eastland Press.

Barral J-P (2008) Has your liver been liberated? TIME Magazine, May 16.

Bertolucci L F (2011) Pandiculation: Nature's way of maintaining the functional integrity of the myofascial system? J Bodyw Mov Ther. July; 15 (3) 268–280.

Chaitow L (ed.) (2014) Fascial Dysfunction: Manual Therapy Approaches. Edinburgh, UK: Handspring Publishing.

Chaudry H, Schleip R, Ji Z et al. (2008) Three-dimensional mathematical model for deformation of human fasciae in manual therapy. J Am Osteopath Assoc. August; 108 (8) 379–390.

Deng L Y and Cheng X (1996) Chinese Acupuncture and Moxibustion, 4th Printing. Foreign Language Press, Beijing, China.

Ernst E (2009) Acupuncture: What does the most reliable evidence tell us? J Pain Symptom Manage. April; 37 (4) 709–714.

Jacobson E (2011) Structural integration: Origins and development. J Altern Complement Med. September; 17 (9) 775–780.

Järvinen T A, Józsa L, Kannus P et al. (2002) Organization and distribution of intramuscular connective tissue in normal and immobilized skeletal muscles. An immunohistochemical polarization and scanning electron microscopic study. J Muscle Res Cell Motil. 23 (3) 245–254.

Juher T F and Pérez E B (2015) An overview of the beneficial effects of hydolysed collagen intake on joint and bone health on skin ageing. Nutr Hosp. July; 32 (Suppl. 1) 62–66.

Kim Y, Hong Y and Park H S (2019) A soft massage tool is advantageous for compressing deep soft tissue with low muscle tension: Therapeutic evidence for self-myofascial release. Complement Ther Med. April; 43, 312–318.

Kjaer M, Langberg H, Heinemeier K et al. (2009) From mechanical loading to collagen synthesis, structural changes and function in human tendon. Scand J Med Sci Sports. August; 19 (4) 500–510.

Kram R and Dawson T J (1998) Energetics and biomechanics of locomotion in red kangaroos (Macropus rufus). Comp Biochem Physiol B Biochem Mol Biol. May; 120 (1) 41–49.

Langevin H M and Yandow J A (2002) Relationship of acupuncture points and meridians to connective tissue planes. Anat Rec. December; 269 (6) 257–265.

Langevin H M, Bouffard N A, Fox J R et al. (2011) Fibroblast cytoskeletal remodeling contributes to connective tissue tension. J Cell Physiol. May; 226 (5) 1166–1175.

Langevin H M, Churchill DL and Cipolla M J (2001) Mechanical signaling through connective tissue: A mechanism for the therapeutic effect of acupuncture. FASEB J. October; 15 (12) 2275–2282.

Langevin H M, Churchill D L, Wu J et al. (2002) Evidence of connective tissue involvement in acupuncture. FASAB J. June; 16 (8) 872–874.

Langevin H M, Konofagou E E, Badger G J et al. (2004) Tissue displacements during acupuncture using ultrasound elastography techniques. Ultrasound Med Biol. September; 30 (9) 1173–1183.

Love R (2011) The Great OOM: The Mysterious Origins of America's First Yogi. London, UK: Penguin Books, pp. 286–287.

Magnusson S P, Langberg H and Kjaer M (2010) The pathogenesis of tendinopathy: Balancing the response to loading. Nat Rev Rheumatol. May; 6 (5) 262–268.

Marr M, Baker J, Lambon N, Perry J and Perry J (2011) The effect of the Bowen technique on hamstring flexibility over time. J Bodyw Mov Ther. July; 15 (3) 281–90.

Meltzer K R, Cao T V, Schad J F et al. (2010) In vitro modeling of repetitive motion injury and myofascial release. J Bodyw Mov Ther. April; 14 (2) 162–171.

Miller J (2021) Clinical foundation and applications for self-myofascial release. In: Lesondak D and Akey A M (eds) Fascia, Function, and Medical Applications. Boca Raton, FL: CRC Press, Chapter 20, pp. 263–274.

Müller D G and Schleip R (2012) Fascial fitness: Suggestions for a fascia-oriented training approach in sports and movement therapies. In: Schleip R, Findley T W, Chaitow L, Huijing P A (eds) Fascia: The Tensional Network of the Human Body. Edinburgh, UK: Elsevier, pp. 467–468.

Myers T W (2020) Anatomy Trains: Myofascial Meridians for Manual Therapists & Movement Professionals, 4th edn. Elsevier, Appendix 4, pp. 339–346.

Najrana T and Sanchez-Esteban J (2016) Mechanotransduction as an adaptation to gravity. Front Pediatr. December; 4, 140.

Rawson E S, Miles M P and Enette Larson-Meyer D (2018) Dietary supplements for health, adaptation, and recovery in athletes. Int J Sport Nutr Exerc Metab. March; 28 (2) 188–199.

Sawicki G S, Lewis C L and Ferris D P (2009) It pays to have a spring in your step. Exerc Sport Sci Rev. July; 37 (3) 130–138.

Schleip R (2012) Plenary lecture, Third International Fascia Research Congress, Vancouver, BC.

Schleip R and Müller D G (2013) Training principles for fascial connective tissues: Scientific foundation and suggested practical application. J Bodyw Mov Ther. January; 17 (1) 103–111.

Servan-Schreiber D (2005) The Instinct to Heal: Curing Depression, Anxiety and Stress Without Drugs and Without Talk Therapy. Emm aus, PA: Rodale Books.

Shah J P and Gilliams E A (2008) Uncovering the biochemical milieu of myofascial trigger points using in vivo microdialysis: An application of muscle pain concepts to myofascial pain syndrome. J Bodyw Mov Ther. October; 12 (4) 371–384.

Staubesand J, Baumbach K U K and Li Y (1997) La structure fine de l'aponévrose jambière. Phlebol. 50 (1) 105–113.

Steffen D and Baar K (2021) Nutrition and loading to improve fascia function. In: Schleip R and Wilke J (eds) Fascia in Sport and Movement, 2nd edn. Edinburgh, UK: Handspring Publishing.

Travell J G (1968) Office Hours: Day and Night: The Autobiography of Janet Travell, M.D. New York, NY: World Publishing Co.

Travell J G and Simons D G (1999a) Myofascial Pain and Dysfunction: The Trigger Point Manual, Volume 1: The Upper Body. Baltimore, MD: Lippincott, Williams & Wilkins.

Travell J G and Simons D G (1999b) Myofascial Pain and Dysfunction: The Trigger Point Manual, Volume 2: The Lower Body. Baltimore, MD: Lippincott, Williams & Wilkins.

Vorselen D, Roos W H, MacKintosh F C et al. (2014) The role of the cytoskeleton in sensing changes in gravity by non-specialized cells. FASEB J. February; 28 (2) 536–547.

Further reading

Avison J (2015) Yoga: Fascia, Anatomy and Movement. Edinburgh, UK: Handspring Publishing.

Barral J-P and Mercier P (2006) Visceral Manipulation, 1st revised edn. Seattle, Washington: Eastland Press.

Clark B (2012) The Complete Guide to Yin Yoga: The Philosophy and Practice of Yin. Ashland, OR: White Cloud Press.

Earls J (2014) Born to Walk: Myofascial Efficiency and the Body in Movement. Chichester, UK: Lotus Publishing and Berkeley, CA: North Atlantic Books.

Frederick A and Frederick C (2014) Fascial Stretch Therapy™. Edinburgh, UK: Handspring Publishing.

Gawande A (2003) Complications: A Surgeon's Notes on an Imperfect Science. New York, NY: Picador.

Grilley P (2012) Yin Yoga: Principles and Practice, 10th Anniversary edn. Ashland, OR: White Cloud Press.

Langevin H M (2013) The science of stretch. The Scientist. May 1. Available: www.the-scientist.com/?articles.view/articleNo/35301/title/The-Science-of-Stretch [May 18, 2022].

Lesondak D and Akey A M (eds) (2021) Fascia, Function, and Medical Applications. Boca Raton, FL: CRC Press.

Miller J (2014) The Roll Model: A Step-by-Step Guide to Erase Pain, Improve Mobility, and Live Better in Your Body. Las Vegas, NV: Victory Belt Press.

Pflugradt S (2022) What really happens to your body when you take collagen? Available: www.livestrong.com/article/13729772-benefits-of-collagen [May 16, 2022].

Powers S (2009) Insight Yoga. Boston, MA: Shambhala Publications.

Rolf I P (1989) Rolfing: Reestablishing the Natural Alignment and Structural Integration of the Human Body for Vitality and Well-Being. Rochester, VT: Healing Arts Press.

Schleip R and Wilke J (eds) (2021) Fascia in Sport and Movement, 2nd edn. Edinburgh, UK: Handspring Publishing.

Street V P (2014) Janet Travell, M.D.: White House Physician and Trigger Point Pioneer. Blurb.

AFTERWORD by Thomas W. Findley

Fascia is both tissue and a system. There are many structures within this overarching concept. For example, the aortic valve, the cardiac arteries, the myocardium and the atrium are different structures in the heart. To describe a new treatment's effects on "the heart" without specifying which structure, or which function (e.g., ejection fraction) limits our understanding and greatly hampers further development of that treatment. We need to specify just which fascial structure or function we mean, more than just "fascia" (Langevin & Huijing 2009).

Here's some additional fascial food for thought, chapter by chapter.

Chapter 1. Fascia is not isotropic. It has different properties when pulled in different directions. Layers of fascia show fibers running in parallel directions, much like reinforcing fibers in packing tape. An angle of 55 degrees to the layer underneath is found in humans, cows, and goats (as well as your garden hose, to contain pressure while remaining flexible). Other angles serve other purposes. Is it possible that we could deduce the function from the angle of the fibers? Nonetheless, we definitely need to rethink how the body is structured, with fascia in mind.

Chapter 2. Our bones are not the only structures which resist compression. We also have microtubules within the cells, and sealed fascial compartments like the ubiquitous bubble wrap packing. The "fascial organ" consists of a body-wide tensional network of fascia. There is a continuity of fibrils from the extracellular matrix through the integrin receptor and the cell membrane to the nucleus. Manual massage after exercise activates the force-conducting pathways to the nucleus, followed within hours by changes in gene transcription (Crane et al. 2012). It is a useful concept to think of the body as a fascial network with connections to muscles and bones, rather than the more traditional view of a musculoskeletal system with fascial connections.

Chapter 3. Energy storage in tissues around the shoulder allows the human to throw at speeds over 100 miles an hour, compared to 20 miles per hour in primates. Precontraction of the muscle stretches connective tissues, which then explosively release to accomplish a movement for which muscle power alone would be insufficient. The storage is diffused across a network of as yet undefined tissues, but the "wind up" for the baseball pitch indicates the whole body is involved.

Chapter 4. The continuum of fascia throughout the body allows it to serve as a body-wide mechanosensitive signaling system, with an important role in proprioception. Muscle spindles concentrate in areas of force transmission to the fascia surrounding the muscle, and contain within them small muscle fibers which can adjust their length in order to be more, or less, responsive to stretch.

Chapter 5. Information is then conducted to the brain, by sensory fibers at speeds from 2 to 100 meters/second, or as mechanical vibrations in the fascia at the speed of sound of 1,500 meters/second.

Chapter 6. Loose connective tissue harbors 15 liters of interstitial fluid. Tension on dermal fibers which surround the hydrophilic ground substance of the extracellular matrix prevent its osmotic pressure from drawing fluid out of the capillary. When these fibers relax, this allows the glycosaminoglycan ground substance to expand and take up fluid. Within minutes after injury, fluid flow out of the capillary can increase 100 fold, causing edema.

Muscle contraction within a thick, resistant fascia layer increases the pressure within this compartment, and squeezes blood and lymphatic fluid against gravity towards the heart as well as raising the contractile efficiency of other muscles in this compartment by 15 per cent. The tight body suits used by swimmers are based on this principle.

Chapters 7 and 8 take us quickly to the forefront of what we know, which remains limited by our ability to describe specifics of fascial diagnosis and treatment. What forces do we apply – stretch, compression, shear, twist, oscillation or vibration? In what direction? Are these forces short or sustained? Are we aiming for immediate tissue change, or change in proprioception, or both? Do we foster repair, remodeling and rebuilding for a future benefit? Are we treating structure or function? Is our aim to reduce the chance of future injury?

Athletes look to exercise physiologists and trainers to improve their performance, and avoid injury. They find that to improve performance in a specific activity (as opposed to strength in an isolated muscle), the best training is that activity itself, which involves motion of the whole body.

Which returns us to fascia as a system as well as a structure.

Tom Findley

Montclair, New Jersey

June 2017

References

Crane J D, Ogborn D I, Cupido C et al (2012) Massage therapy attenuates inflammatory signaling after exercise-induced muscle damage. Sci Transl Med. February; 4 (119) 119ra13.

Langevin H M and Huijing P A (2009) Communicating about fascia: History, pitfalls, and recommendations. Int J Ther Massage Bodywork. December; 2 (4) 3–8.

AFTERWORD by Sasha Chaitow

In this book David Lesondak has provided a rare roadmap to the current state of fascia research and its implications, accessible to newcomers, clinicians, and scientists alike. Setting it apart from other titles is the sheer interdisciplinary scope of the work already done and the manifold applications of this growing understanding of the fascial network.

The neuroscientific, interoceptive, and internal implications alone are staggering, with significant potential for the current scientific interest in the connections between physical and mental health. Understanding fascia reveals the interconnectedness of the body's systems in a way that has not been available to science before, providing a blueprint for new lines of interdisciplinary collaboration with the potential to revolutionize our understanding of health and disease processes and develop truly multimodal therapeutic approaches to a range of conditions. This is in keeping with the conceptual framework underlying the current paradigm shift towards whole-person health care, for if the organism is shaped and governed by a biotensegral matrix, the most appropriate way to address it can only be through a matrix of minds and specialties that reflects its multifactorial and interconnected nature. The future seems rich with possibility and, with the help of this book, the maturing state of fascia research is now in a position to attract engagement from multiple medical disciplines.

For this potential to be fulfilled, key milestones require attention. Despite the multidisciplinary input into fascia *research*, engagement with and application of that research has until now been largely skewed towards those disciplines dealing with musculoskeletal dysfunction and rehabilitation, manual therapy, and/or performance optimization. This broad cluster of professions includes osteopaths – for whom the potential of fascia has been a core principle since the foundation of the profession – physiotherapists, chiropractors, athletic trainers, massage therapists, and a kaleidoscope of other bodywork professions. These related but distinct disciplines have issues of their own to contend with, including matters of interprofessional communication and nomenclature, heterogeneity in the size, quality, and application of the evidence base, regulation, education, scope, locus, and nature of practice, and often widely differing philosophical principles. This diversity has sparked the multiple applications and branded "modalities" some of which are noted in Chapter 8 of this book, bringing fascia-oriented therapies into broader application. However, this situation is fraught with difficulty, as eagerness for practical applications overshadows and overtakes the slow, meticulous process that is scientific research, often producing a host of misconceptions and further fragmentation of an already heterogeneous array of clinical approaches.

In recent years some organizations have attempted to bridge the practitioner–researcher divide, though these efforts have often fallen short of expectations. At the time of writing, however (May 2022), the International Consortium on Manual Therapies has developed working groups and discussion groups organized by profession, flattening the hierarchy of the research–clinician spectrum, and early reports from its inaugural conference suggest that this formula is beginning to bear fruit.

The research–practitioner divide is defined by wholly different educational foundations and objectives. Most practitioners lack training and skills in experimental methods, research conventions, and research literacy, and this is as true for graduates of four-year programs as of vocational training, as these skills are simply not prioritized in the curricula, and it falls to haphazard continuing professional development/education courses to fill the gap. Unfortunately, these do not tend to be subject to rigorous regulation and therefore the quality of the training can be hit and miss, largely governed by the laws of free market competition and good publicity rather than merit. The same applies to the many branded techniques offered by private practitioners in some regions. This phenomenon has led to fractures within these communities, with ideology replacing the weaknesses in critical appraisal skills, and sometimes heated debates clouding the key issue: That there is not sufficient evidence for some practices. This is not the same as negative evidence, and improved training is needed in research literacy, critical thinking skills, and achieving the fine balance between the three "legs" of the biopsychosocial model.

Meanwhile, laboratory researchers are frequently unaware of the issues that practitioners contend with, and what they do and encounter in the clinical setting, or indeed the wider context and debates regarding validation. As a result, the research produced and reported frequently fails to translate into applicable clinical terms or to begin explaining the all-important mechanisms of action that are necessary for a robust evidence base. In the case of fascia, great inroads have been made as evidenced by this very book, but simultaneously this has led to what some see as an overzealous uptake and promotion of "fascial" therapies with the most tenuous of scientific foundations (due to the lack of research literacy mentioned previously), driven more by commercial and personal ambition. This has then provoked reactions that dismiss the significance of fascia as hype, overlooking the very robust research that this book so effectively

presents. It is the case that sometimes this idea of "translational research" is misinterpreted as meaning that every research study ought to have a practical dimension that practitioners can immediately transfer into their technique. This is a misperception; translational research may involve mechanisms of action, comparative benefit and cost-effectiveness and consideration of the relative value of a given therapeutic protocol in the context of a multimodal regimen. It is equally crucial, as the emphasis on evidence-informed practice within the biopsychosocial model continues to grow, for patient preference and the sociology of medical practice from both clinician and patient perspectives to be included in the areas of inquiry. There is also an urgency for educationalists and school-owners across this professional spectrum to tackle these matters in concert, addressing the gaps in education, clinical reasoning skills, and higher order inquiry that would provide a welcome antidote to the aforementioned phenomena.

A serious consequence of not tackling these issues is the continued reputational damage of otherwise valuable and respectable allied health professions, and the repercussions on the end-users; the patients. Historically many of these practices derived from the sphere of so-called "alternative," (later "complementary," now "integrative" or "functional") medicine, which self-defined as a distinct approach to healthcare in opposition to "allopathic," or conventional bio-medicine. It has taken decades to uproot the truly pseudoscientific elements of these professions, to improve training, regulation, and achieve forms of validation that ensure quality standards for these professions. Yet the damage of "guilt by association" persists strongly even among practitioners of the same professions, with partisanship marring what might otherwise be fruitful ground for progress. Meanwhile, biomedicine has begun to welcome the more holistic approach underpinning whole-person care, and statistics suggest that a majority of medical physicians are positively inclined towards many integrative techniques, particularly where appropriate guidelines for practice within multimodal care teams have been introduced. Therefore, it is even more crucial that educational leaders and communication spokespeople within the broader fields of bodywork and movement therapies explore the options for building bridges for multidisciplinary collaboration, as David Lesondak has personally been able to do, resulting in enthusiastic reception and interest among biomedical professionals.

Some may wonder what the preceding paragraphs have to do with fascia; I am certain I will be forgiven for emphasizing that *it is all connected* in something closely resembling a biotensegrity structure where function does, to an extent, dictate form, even as pulling any one strand distorts the whole. There is no linearity to the research–education–practice–communication paradigm. As previously noted, important initiatives are evolving to address the individual issues, but in the meantime, all of the strands in this complex structure require realignment with the recognition that each is contingent on all others.

This may be achieved with simultaneous actions along the following lines, which should be perceived as the moving parts of an interdependent whole where researchers might be compared to neural centers; educators to circulatory functions; and clinicians to single cells. Science communicators, broadly defined, are the connective tissue.

- **Basic science researchers:** All too often, researchers are deeply immersed in their direct laboratory activities, or focused on seeking funding followed by publication. This creates a silo that is difficult to break out of, especially if they are not aware of the scale and complexity of the issues. Balance may be found by seeking out clinician communities, participating in practice-focused conferences and relevant working groups both formally and informally, but outside the lab.

- **Social science and humanities researchers:** Unlike medical education, allied health education and practice profiles are not well researched (with the exception of osteopathic medicine). This information is critical to addressing some of the issues outlined above. Due to their key transferable skills, humanities scholars are already working alongside medical educationalists and establishing curricula to improve a range of higher order thinking skills of direct relevance to both research literacy and clinical practice. There is much fertile ground for collaborating with both educators and researchers to improve matters on both sides of the spectrum.

- **Allied/integrative/functional educators:** Though isolated voices and significant thought leaders have been calling for improved nomenclature, quality standards, and educational rigor for years, there is much fragmentation and little concerted effort in this direction. Awareness of the sociological framework impacting education, along with recent developments in biomedical education, may provide a valuable roadmap for closer collaboration with colleagues in this area.

- **Allied/integrative/functional health clinicians:** The key issues have been addressed in the main body of this afterword. Professional attention to these through honest self-assessment regarding weaknesses in critical skills, research literacy and awareness as well as a candid appraisal of trends, fads, branding, and commercialization compared to deeper engagement with the skills deficits described would raise the level of dialogue significantly, offering personal and professional benefit.

- **Biomedical educationalists and clinicians:** Given the established shift towards whole-person practice, biomedicine has much to gain from closer collaboration with the holistic allied health professions, both at levels of leadership as well as individual practice, in a spirit of collegial collaboration that ultimately benefits patients seeking care. Each can provide the other with important know-how and perspectives, but a common language is needed because of the different value systems involved. The inclusion of social science scholars, humanities scholars, and science communicators in this work would be greatly valuable.

- **Science communicators:** (including educators, clinical librarians, science writers): As a member of this category, I have few illusions as to the challenges of acquiring an accurate overview and familiarity with the complexity of concepts and issues involved. The responsibility of being the individual tasked with communicating accurately among is significant (reminiscent of the role of fibroblasts). Even if science communicators are specialized in one or other area, it is critical that they should have a range of transferable skills, and

not be professionally invested in one or other clinical profession to the degree that this may cloud their impartiality. These are the people who are in a position to contribute the most to building the bridges between the other strands of the whole, but it requires a good understanding of the issues and concerns involved in each layer.

The great value of this book, and its author's experience, is that it allows readers from any of these backgrounds to discover how deeply significant fascia and its research is to our understanding of the whole human organism, and its implication for every level of health care. It is eagerly hoped that through a fresh perception of the impact of this interconnectivity of human endeavor, solutions will be implemented to revolutionize and unite the health professions for mutual benefit, and most importantly, for public health.

Sasha Chaitow PhD

Corfu

May 2022

Department of Physiotherapy

School of Health Rehabilitation Sciences

University of Patras (Greece)

Series Editor

The Leon Chaitow Library of Bodywork and Movement Therapies

GLOSSARY

These are terms used in fascia research and taken from the Fascia Research Congress.

actin is a common protein found in many eukaryotic cell types. It polymerizes forming microfilaments that have an array of functions including regulating contractility, motility, cytokinesis, phagocytosis, adhesion, cell morphology, and providing structural support.

adhesions are bands of scar-like tissue that form between two surfaces inside the body.

adhesive capsulitis is an inflammatory condition that restricts motion in the shoulder, commonly referred to as "frozen shoulder."

alpha-1-antitrypsin is a glycoprotein, generally known as a serum trypsin inhibitor, that inhibits a wide variety of proteases. It protects tissues from enzymes of inflammatory cells, especially elastase, and the concentration can rise upon acute inflammation. In its absence, elastase is free to break down elastin.

alpha smooth muscle actin is an isoform typical of smooth muscle cells and one of six known types of actin. In addition to its presence in organ tissue, alpha smooth muscle actin has been identified in myofibroblasts where it plays an important role in focal adhesion maturation and inhibition of cell motility.

aponeurosis is a thin, flat tendon-like expansion of fascia important in the attachment of muscles to bones and other muscles and in the formation of sheaths around muscles.

apoptosis is a morphologic pattern of cell death affecting single cells, marked by shrinkage of the cell, condensation of chromatin, formation of cytoplasmic blebs, and fragmentation of the cell into membrane-bound apoptotic bodies that are eliminated by phagocytosis. It is a mechanism for cell deletion in the regulation of cell populations.

astrocytes are a neuroglial cell of ectodermal origin, characterized by fibrous, protoplasmic, or plasmatofibrous processes. Collectively, such cells are called astroglia.

ATP is adenosine triphosphate, an adenosine-derived nucleotide that supplies large amounts of energy to cells for various biochemical processes, including muscle contraction and sugar metabolism.

basal lamina is the layer of the basement membrane lying next to the basal surface of the adjoining cell layer, composed of an electron-dense lamina densa and an electron-lucent lamina lucida.

basement membrane is a sheet of amorphous extracellular material upon which the basal surfaces of epithelial cells rest; other cells associated with basement membranes are muscle cells, Schwann cells, fat cells, and capillaries. The membrane is interposed between the cellular elements and the underlying connective tissue. It comprises two layers, the basal lamina and the reticular lamina, and is composed of Type IV collagen (which is unique to basement membranes), laminin, fibronectin, and heparan sulfate proteoglycans.

benign joint hypermobility syndrome is an alternate name for Ehlers-Danlos syndrome, type 3 inherited as an autosomal dominant trait and characterized by hypermobility of the joints with minimal abnormalities of the skin.

bradykinin is a nonapeptide produced by activation of the kinin system in a variety of inflammatory conditions. It is a potent vasodilator and also increases vascular permeability, stimulates pain receptors, and causes contraction of a variety of extravascular smooth muscles.

calcitonin gene-related peptide is a 37-amino acid polypeptide encoded by the calcitonin gene that acts as a potent vasodilator and neurotransmitter. It is widely distributed in the central and peripheral nervous systems and is also present in the adrenal medulla and gastrointestinal tract.

caldesmon is a protein that exists in two isoforms: a high molecular weight form found in smooth muscles that can bind to actin and tropomyosin, prevent actin-myosin linkage, and inhibit muscle contraction; and a low molecular weight form found in non-muscle tissue and cells that plays a role in regulating the microfilament network.

capsaicin is an alkaloid irritating to the skin and mucous membranes. It is the pungent active principle in capsicum (cayenne), used as a topical counterirritant and analgesic.

cartilage is a specialized, fibrous connective tissue, forming most of the temporary skeleton of the embryo, providing a model in which most of the bones develop, and constituting an important part of the growth mechanism of the organism. It exists in several types, the most important of which are hyaline cartilage, elastic cartilage, and fibrocartilage.

cell migration is a central process in the development and maintenance of multicellular organisms. Tissue formation during embryonic development, wound healing and immune responses all require the orchestrated movement of cells in a particular direction to a specific location.

cell signaling is the process by which a cell receives and acts on some external chemical or physical signal, such as a hormone, including receiving the information at specific receptors in the plasma membrane, conveying the signal across the plasma membrane into the cell, and subsequently inducing an intracellular chain of other signaling molecules, thereby stimulating a specific cellular response.

chondroblasts are immature cartilage cells which produce the cartilaginous matrix.

collagen is an abundant protein that constitutes a major component of fascia, giving it strength and flexibility. At least 14 types exist, each composed of tropocollagen units that share a common triple-helical shape but that vary somewhat in composition between types, with the types being localized to different tissues, stages, or functions. In some types, including the most common, Type I, the tropocollagen rods associate to form fibrils or fibers; in other types the rods are not fibrillar but are associated with fibrillar collagens, while in others they form non-fibrillar, nonperiodic but structured networks.

collagenoblasts are cells that arise from fibroblasts and, as they mature, are associated with the production of collagen. They form cartilage and bone by metaplasia and proliferate at sites of chronic inflammation.

compartment syndrome involves the compression of nerves and blood vessels within a fascial compartment. This leads to impaired blood flow and muscle and nerve damage.

connexin is the primary protein component of connexon, the functional unit of a gap junction.

creep refers to the time-dependent tendency of a tissue to deform permanently as a result of application and maintenance of a stress at a set level.

cytokines are a generic term for non-antibody proteins released by one cell population (e.g., primed T lymphocytes) on contact with specific antigens, which act as intercellular mediators, as in the generation of an immune response.

cytoskeleton is the conspicuous internal reinforcement in the cytoplasm of a cell, consisting of tonofibrils, terminal web, or other microfilaments.

deep fascia is the dense fibrous fascia that interpenetrates and surrounds the muscles, bones, nerves, and blood vessels of the body.

deformation is the process of adapting in shape or form, as when erythrocytes change in shape as they pass through capillaries. In dysmorphology, deformation refers to a type of structural defect characterized by the abnormal form or position of a body part, caused by a nondisruptive mechanical force.

differentiated myofibroblast describes a myofibroblast that is capable of expressing alpha smooth muscle actin.

Ehlers-Danlos syndrome is a group of inherited disorders of the connective tissue, occurring in at least ten types, based on clinical, genetic, and biochemical evidence, varying in severity from mild to lethal, and transmitted genetically as autosomal recessive, autosomal dominant, or X-linked recessive traits. The major manifestations include hyperextensible skin and joints, easy bruisability, friability of tissues with bleeding and poor wound healing, calcified subcutaneous spheroids, and pseudotumors. Variably present in some types are cardiovascular, gastrointestinal, orthopedic, and ocular defects.

elastin is a yellow scleroprotein, the essential constituent of yellow elastic connective tissue. It is brittle when dry, but when moist is flexible and elastic.

electron microscopy is an imaging technique that uses electrons to illuminate and create an image of a specimen. It has much higher magnification and resolving power than a light microscope, with magnifications up to about two million times compared to about two thousand, allowing it to see smaller objects and greater detail in these objects. Unlike a light microscope, which uses glass lenses to focus light, the electron microscope uses electrostatic and electromagnetic lenses to control the illumination and imaging of the specimen.

endomysium is the fascial layer that ensheaths single muscle fibers.

endoneurium is the innermost fascial layer of a peripheral nerve, forming an interstitial layer around each individual fiber outside the neurilemma.

endotenon is a thin fascial membrane within a tendon that invests each collagen fibril, each collagen fiber, and envelops the primary, secondary, and tertiary fiber bundles together.

endothelium is the layer of epithelial cells that lines the cavities of the heart, the lumina of blood and lymph vessels, and the serous cavities of the body.

enkephalins are either of two simple pentapeptides that function as neurotransmitters or neuromodulators at many locations in the brain and spinal cord and play a part in pain perception, movement, mood, behavior, and neuroendocrine regulation. They are also found in nerve plexuses and exocrine glands of the gastrointestinal tract.

eosinophilic fasciitis is an inflammation of the fasciae of the extremities, associated with eosinophilia, edema, and swelling. The etiology is unknown but it frequently occurs following strenuous exercise. Also called Shulman's syndrome.

epimysium is the fascial layer which envelops an entire muscle.

epineurium is the outermost fascial layer of a peripheral nerve, surrounding the entire nerve and containing its supplying blood vessels and lymphatics.

epitenon is a fine, loose connective tissue sheath covering a tendon over its entire length.

extracellular matrix refers to any material produced by cells and excreted to the extracellular space within the tissues. It takes the form of both ground substance and fibers and is composed chiefly of fibrous elements, proteins involved in cell adhesion, and glycosaminoglycans and other molecules. It serves as a scaffolding holding tissues together and its form and composition help determine tissue characteristics. In epithelia, it includes the basement membrane.

fascia is the soft tissue component of the connective tissue system. It interpenetrates and surrounds muscles, bones, organs, nerves, blood vessels, and other structures. Fascia is an uninterrupted, three-dimensional web of tissue that extends from head to toe, from front to back, from interior to exterior. It is responsible for maintaining structural integrity; for providing support and protection; and acts as a shock absorber. Fascia has an essential role in hemodynamic and biochemical processes, and provides the matrix that allows for intercellular communication. After injury, it is the fascia that creates an environment for tissue repair. Fascia can refer to dense planar fascial sheets (such as the fascia lata) as well as joint capsules, organ capsules, muscular septa, ligaments, retinacula, aponeuroses, tendons, myofascia, neurofascia, and other fibrous collagenous tissues.

fasciacyte is a fibroblast-like cell that produces hyaluronan (HA) which is essential for proper fascial gliding.

fasciagenic describes a condition that originates in or is caused by the fascia.

fasciotomy is a surgical incision or transection of fascia, often performed to release pressure in compartment syndrome.

fibroblasts are flat elongated fascial cells with cytoplasmic processes at each end, having a flat, oval, vesicular nucleus. Fibroblasts, which differentiate into chondroblasts, collagenoblasts, osteoblasts, and myofibroblasts, form the fibrous tissues in the body, including tendons, aponeuroses, supporting and binding tissues of all sorts.

fibromyalgia is a common chronic rheumatic syndrome characterized by widespread pain in fibrous tissues, muscles, tendons, and other connective tissues, resulting in painful muscles without weakness. The cause of this disorder is unknown, but poor sleep quality seems to be an important factor in its pathogenesis.

fibronectins are any of several related adhesive glycoproteins. One form circulates in plasma, acting as an opsonin; another is a cell-surface protein that mediates cellular adhesive interactions. Fibronectins are important in fascia, where they crosslink to collagen, and are also involved in aggregation of platelets.

fibronexus is an adhesion in a myofibroblast that links actin across the cell membrane to molecules in the extracellular-matrix-like fibronectin and collagen.

fibrosis is the formation of fibrous tissue, as in repair or replacement of parenchymatous elements.

gap junctions are a type of intercellular junction comprising a narrowed portion (about 3 nm) of the intercellular space that contains channels or pores composed of hexagonal arrays of membrane-spanning proteins around a central lumen (connexon) through which pass ions and small molecules such as most sugars, amino acids, nucleotides, vitamins, hormones, and cyclic AMP. In electrically excitable tissues, these gap junctions serve to transmit electrical impulses via ionic currents and are known as electrotonic synapses.

glycosaminoglycans are any of several high molecular weight linear heteropolysaccharides having disaccharide repeating units containing an N-acetylhexosamine and a hexose or hexuronic acid; either or both residues may be sulfated. This class of compounds includes the chondroitin sulfates, dermatan sulfates, heparan sulfate and heparin, keratan sulfates, and hyaluronic acid. All except heparin occur in proteoglycans.

Golgi receptors are mechanosensory receptors found in dense proper fascia, in ligaments (Golgi end organs), in joint capsules, as well as around myotendinous junctions (Golgi tendon organs).

goniometer is a tool which measures a joint's axis and range of motion.

granulation tissue is the perfused connective tissue matrix that replaces a fibrin clot in wound healing. The extracellular matrix of granulation tissue is created and modified by fibroblasts.

hyaluronan is a glycosaminoglycan that is part of the extracellular matrix of synovial fluid, vitreous humor, cartilage, blood vessels, skin, and the umbilical cord. Along with lubricin, it maintains viscosity of the extracellular matrix allowing for necessary lubrication of certain tissues.

hyaluronic acid see **hyaluronan**

hypermobility refers to a greater than normal range of motion in a joint, which may occur naturally in otherwise normal persons or may be a sign of joint instability. Also known as laxity.

hypertonia refers to excessive tone of the skeletal muscles that increases their resistance to passive stretching.

hypertrophy is the enlargement or overgrowth of an organ or part due to an increase in size of its constituent cells.

hysteresis is a property of systems that do not instantly react to the forces applied to them, but react slowly, or do not return completely to their original state.

integrins refer to any of a family of heterodimeric cell-adhesion receptors, consisting of two non-covalently linked polypeptide chains, designated α and β, that mediate cell-to-cell and cell-to-extracellular-matrix interactions.

interleukin is a generic term for a group of multifunctional cytokines that are produced by a variety of lymphoid and nonlymphoid cells and have effects at least partly within the lymphopoietic system; originally believed to be produced chiefly by and to act chiefly upon leukocytes.

interstitial fluid is the extracellular fluid that bathes the cells of most tissues but which is not within the confines of the blood or lymph vessels and is not a transcellular fluid. It is formed by filtration through the blood capillaries and is drained away as lymph. It is the extracellular fluid volume minus the lymph volume, the plasma volume, and the transcellular fluid volume.

kinins are proteins in the blood that influence certain muscle contractions, affect blood pressure (especially hypotension or low blood pressure), increase blood flow throughout the body, increase the permeability of small capillaries, and stimulate pain receptors.

lamellipodia are delicate sheet-like extensions of cytoplasm which form transient adhesions with the cell substrate and wave gently, enabling the cell to move along the substrate.

laminin is an adhesive glycoprotein component of the basement membrane. It binds to heparan sulfate, Type IV collagen, and specific cell-surface receptors and is involved in the attachment of epithelial cells to underlying connective tissue.

ligament is a band of fascia that connects bones or supports viscera. Some ligaments are distinct fibrous structures; some are folds of fascia or of indurated peritoneum; still others are relics of fetal vessels or organs.

lysyl oxidase-like protein 1 is an enzyme responsible for elastin crosslinking and a close homolog of lysyl oxidase. It plays a significant role in directing enzymatic deposition onto elastic fibers by mediating interactions with tropoelastin. It is associated with extracellular matrix remodeling during active fibrotic disorders and in the early stromal reaction of breast cancer.

Marfan syndrome is a disorder of connective tissue which causes skeletal defects typically recognized in a tall, lanky person. A person with Marfan syndrome may exhibit long limbs and spider-like fingers, chest abnormalities, curvature of the spine and a particular set of facial features including a highly arched palate, and crowded teeth.

mechanoreceptors are sensory receptors that respond to mechanical pressure or deformation.

They include Pacinian corpuscles, Meissner's corpuscles, Merkel's discs, Ruffini corpuscles, and some interstitial nerve endings.

mechanotransduction is the mechanism by which cells convert mechanical stimulus into chemical activity.

mepyramine is an antihistaminic pharmacological substance frequently used as an in vitro contractile agent for tissues containing myofibroblasts.

morphogenesis is the evolution and development of form, as in the development of the shape of a particular organ or part of the body.

morphometric analysis is a method of extracting measurements from shapes to study the "form follows function" aspect of biology, mapping the changes in an organism's shape in regards to its function.

myofascial pain syndrome is a chronic musculoskeletal pain disorder associated with local or referred pain, decreased range of motion, autonomic phenomena, local twitch response in the affected muscle, and muscle weakness without atrophy.

myofibroblasts are atypical fibroblasts that combine the ultra-structural features of both fibroblasts and smooth muscle cells. Due to their expression of stress fiber bundles containing alpha smooth muscle actin and due to strengthened adhesion sites on their membrane, these cells possess a much higher contractile potential than normal fibroblasts.

myosin is the most abundant protein in muscle, occurring chiefly in the A band. Along with actin, it is responsible for the contraction and relaxation of muscle. Myosin has enzymatic properties, acting as an ATPase. It is the main constituent of the thick filaments of muscle fibers.

neuromatrix is a hypothesized network of neurons in the brain that, in addition to responding to sensory stimulation, could continuously generate a neurosignature, a characteristic pattern of impulses indicating that the body is intact and unequivocally one's own.

neuropathy is a functional disturbance or pathological change in the peripheral nervous system.

neuroplasticity refers to the changes that occur in the organization of the brain as a result of experience.

nociceptors are receptors for pain that are activated by physical, mechanical, thermal, electrical, or chemical stimuli.

osteoblasts are cells that arise from fibroblasts and are associated with the production of bone.

osteogenesis imperfecta is a congenital disease caused by a genetic defect that affects Type I collagen and results in extremely fragile bones. Also called brittle bone disease.

oxytocin is a nonapeptide secreted by the magnocellular neurons of the hypothalamus and stored in the neurohypophysis along with vasopressin. It promotes uterine contractions and milk ejection, contributes to the second stage of labor, and is released during orgasm in both sexes. In the brain, oxytocin regulates circadian homeostasis, such as body temperature, activity level, and wakefulness and is involved in social recognition, bonding, and trust formation.

Pacinian corpuscles are lamellar or lamellated large encapsulated nerve endings located in fascia that are sensitive to pressure, vibration, and acceleration of movement.

perimysium is the fascial membrane which groups individual muscle fibers (between 10 to 100+) into bundles or fascicles.

perineurium is an intermediate layer of fascia in a peripheral nerve, surrounding each bundle (fasciculus) of nerve fibers.

peritenon is the outer fascial layer of a tendon in tendons that are contained within a synovial sheath.

Peyronie's disease is a fascial thickening that deforms the penis, distorting the shape of an erection.

piezoelectric is the ability of some materials to generate an electric potential in response to applied mechanical stress.

plantar fasciitis refers to an inflammatory condition of the plantar fascia.

plantar fibromatosis refers to the formation of fibrous, tumor-like nodules arising from the deep layer of the plantar fascia, manifested as single or multiple nodular swellings, sometimes accompanied by pain but is usually unassociated with contractures.

pressure algometer is an instrument that measures mechanical nociceptive thresholds.

prestress is endogenous tension.

procollagen is the precursor molecule of collagen, synthesized in the fibroblast, osteoblast, etc., and cleaved to form collagen extracellularly.

proprioception is perception mediated by sensory nerve endings found in muscles and fascia, which give information concerning movement and position of the body.

proteoglycans are polysaccharide-proteins that are found in the extracellular matrix of fascia, composed mainly of polysaccharide chains, particularly glycosaminoglycans, as well as minor protein components that form large complexes, both to other proteoglycans, to hyaluronan and to fibrous matrix proteins (such as collagen). They are also involved in binding cations (such as sodium, potassium and calcium) and water and also regulating the movement of molecules through the matrix. Evidence also shows they can affect the activity and stability of proteins and signaling molecules within the matrix.

proto-myofibroblasts are myofibroblasts that do not contain alpha smooth muscle actin, but can be distinguished from fibroblasts by the presence of stress fibers.

pseudopodium is a temporary cytoplasmic extrusion by means of which an ameba or other ameboid organism or cell moves about or engulfs food. Pseudopodia are of four types: axopodia, filopodia, lobopodia, and reticulopodia.

reticular fibers are fascial fibers composed of collagen Type III that form the reticular framework of lymphoid and myeloid tissue and also occur in the interstitial tissue of glandular organs, the papillary layer of the skin, and elsewhere.

retinaculum is a thickened band of fascia that retains an organ or tissue in place.

Ruffini endings are a type of lamellated corpuscle that are slowly adapting receptors for sensations of continuous pressure.

sclerosis is an induration or hardening caused by inflammation, fascial thickening, or disease of the interstitial fluid.

serotonin is a monoamine vasoconstrictor, synthesized in the intestinal chromaffin cells or in central or peripheral neurons and found in high concentrations in many body tissues, including the intestinal mucosa, pineal body, and central nervous system.

spasmodic torticollis refers to intermittent dystonia and spasms of the cervical muscles, particularly the sternocleidomastoid and trapezius. This results in distorted posture, exhibited by a twisting of the neck and an unnatural position of the head. Also called wry neck.

substance P is a short-chain polypeptide that functions as a neurotransmitter and as a neuromodulator.

superficial fascia is comprised mainly of loose areolar connective tissue and adipose tissue and is the layer that primarily determines the shape of a body. In addition to its subcutaneous presence, this type of fascia surrounds organs and glands, neurovascular bundles, and is found at many other locations.

tendon is a fibrous cord of fascia by which a muscle is attached.

tendon sheath is a membranous sleeve which envelops the tendon and creates a lubricated low-friction environment for easy movement.

tensegrity is the property of materials made strong by the unison of tensioned and compressed parts.

thixotropy is the property of a material to show a time-dependent change in viscosity. The longer it is subjected to shear forces, the lower its viscosity.

transdifferentiation is a biological process that occurs when a non-stem cell transforms into a different type of cell, or when an already differentiated stem cell creates cells outside its already established differentiation.

transforming growth factor refers to any of several proteins secreted by transformed cells and stimulating growth of normal cells, although not causing transformation. TGF-α binds the epidermal growth factor receptor and also stimulates growth of microvascular endothelial cells. TGF-β exists as several subtypes, all of which are found in hematopoietic tissue, stimulate wound healing, and in vitro are antagonists of lymphopoiesis and myelopoiesis.

tropocollagen is the basic structural unit of collagen; a helical structure consisting of three polypeptide chains, each chain composed of about a thousand amino acids, coiled around each other to form a spiral and stabilized by inter- and intra-chain covalent bonds. It is rich in glycine, proline, hydroxyproline, and hydroxylysine; the last two rarely occur in other proteins.

tropoelastin is the precursor of elastin.

tropomyosin, along with troponin, regulates the shortening of the muscle protein filaments actin and myosin. In the absence of nerve impulses to muscle fibers, tropomyosin blocks interaction between myosin crossbridges and actin filaments.

ultrasound elastography is a noninvasive imaging method to measure stiffness or strain of soft tissue or to provide images of tissue morphology or other biomechanical information.

vacuoles refer to any small space or cavity formed in the protoplasm of a cell.

vimentin filaments are intermediate filaments of the cytoskeleton that are responsible for maintaining cell integrity. They act as cytoskeletal support structures, play a role in mitosis, and are clustered particularly around the nucleus, probably helping to control its location. In cells containing more than one type of intermediate filament, vimentin filaments are always present.

viscoelastic describes materials that exhibit both viscous and elastic characteristics when undergoing plastic deformation. Viscous materials, like honey, resist shear flow and strain linearly with time when a stress is applied. Elastic materials strain instantaneously when stretched and just as quickly return to their original state once the stress is removed. Viscoelastic materials have elements of both of these properties and, as such, exhibit time-dependent strain.

vitronectin is a multifunctional adhesive glycoprotein occurring in serum and various tissues and having binding sites for integrins, collagen, heparin, complement components, and perforin. Its functions include regulation of the coagulation, fibrinolytic, and complement cascades, and it plays a role in hemostasis, wound healing, tissue remodeling, and cancer. It binds plasminogen activator inhibitor; mediates the inflammatory and repair reactions occurring at sites of tissue injury; and promotes adhesion, spreading, and migration of cells.

Wolff's law is the theory developed by nineteenth-century anatomist and surgeon Julius Wolff that states that bone in a healthy person or animal will adapt to the loads it is placed under. If loading on a particular bone increases, the bone will remodel itself over time to become stronger to resist that sort of loading. The converse is true as well: If the loading on a bone decreases, the bone will become weaker due to turnover as it is less metabolically costly to maintain and there is no stimulus for continued remodeling that is required to maintain bone mass.

Figure 1.1 Photo by author. Reproduced with kind permission from Thomas W. Myers.

Figure 1.2 Photo by Nicole Trombley and Rachelle Clauson. Courtesy of AnatomySCAPES.com.

Figure 1.3 Reproduced with permission from Handspring Publishing. Adapted from Stecco A., Stecco C., and Stecco L. (2017) The superficial fascia. In: Liem T., Tozzi P., and Chila A. (eds) (2017) *Fascia in the Osteopathic Field.* Edinburgh, UK: Handspring Publishing.

Figure 1.5 Photo by Nicole Trombley and Rachelle Clauson. Courtesy of AnatomySCAPES.com.

Figure 1.6 Illustration courtesy of fascialnet.com.

Figure 1.9 Illustration courtesy of fascialnet.com.

Figure 1.10 Photo by Robert Strovers, used with kind permission. www.robertstrovers.com.

Figure 1.13 Reproduced with permission from the American Society for Cell Biology. From Jiang H. and Grinnell F. (2005) Cell–matrix entanglement and mechanical anchorage of 24 fibroblasts in three-dimensional collagen matrices. *Molecular Biology of the Cell.* November; 16 (11) 5070–5076.

Figure 1.14 Reprinted by permission of Springer Nature from the *Journal of Muscle Research and Cell Motility.* Organization and distribution of intramuscular connective tissue in normal and immobilized skeletal muscles. An immunohistochemical, polarization and scanning electron microscopic study. Järvinen T. A., Józsa L., Kannus P., Järvinen T. L. N., Järvinen M. 23 (3) 145–154. 2002.

Figure 1.15 Reproduced with the kind permission of Endovivo Productions and J.-C. Guimberteau MD.

Figure 1.16 Reproduced with the kind permission of Endovivo Productions and J.-C. Guimberteau MD.

Figure 1.17 Reproduced with the kind permission of Endovivo Productions and J.-C. Guimberteau MD.

Figure 1.18 Reproduced with the kind permission of Endovivo Productions and J.-C. Guimberteau MD.

Figure 2.4 Illustration by O. C. Marsh, 1896.

Figure 2.5 Photos by Coletta Perry. Reproduced with kind permission.

Figure 2.6 *Early X-Piece*, 1948, wood and nylon. Sculpture by Kenneth Snelson. Reproduced with permission.

Figure 2.7 Kenneth Snelson, the artist in his studio with tensegrity sculpture, 1960. Reproduced with permission.

Figure 2.9 Getty Images.

Figure 2.12 Reproduced with kind permission from Carrie D. Gaynor and Jennifer Wideman.

Figure 2.13 Reproduced with kind permission from Professor Emilia Entcheva.

Figure 2.14 Image courtesy of Paul Emsley and MRC Laboratory of Molecular Biology.

Figure 2.18 Photo by author. Reproduced with kind permission from Thomas W. Myers.

Figure 2.19 Photo by author. Reproduced with kind permission from Thomas W. Myers.

Figure 2.20 Reproduced with permission from Elsevier. From Kassolik K., Andrzejewski W., Brzozowski M. et al. (2013) Comparison of massage based on the tensegrity principle and classic massage in treating chronic shoulder pain. *Journal of Manipulative and Physiological Therapeutics.* September 36 (7) 418–427.

Figure 3.1 Reproduced with kind permission from Thomas W. Myers.

Figure 3.2 Reprinted by permission of Handspring Publishing. From Liem T., Tozzi P., and Chila A. (eds) (2017) *Fascia in the Osteopathic Field.* Edinburgh, UK: Handspring Publishing.

Figure 3.8 Museum of Osteopathic Medicine, Kirksville, Missouri [1980.406.01].

Figure 3.12 Illustration courtesy of fascialnet.com.

Figure 3.13 Reprinted by permission of Springer Nature from the *Journal of Muscle Research and Cell Motility.* The morphology and mechanical properties of endomysium in series-fibred muscles; variations with muscle length. Purslow, P.P., Trotter, J.A., 15 (3) 299–304. 1994.

Figure 3.14 Reprinted by permission of Springer Nature from the *Journal of Muscle Research and Cell Motility.* The morphology and mechanical

properties of endomysium in series-fibred muscles; variations with muscle length. Purslow, P.P., Trotter, J.A., 15 (3) 299–304. 1994.

Figure 3.15 From "Muscle Attitudes" DVD. Reproduced with the kind permission of Endovivo Productions and J.-C. Guimberteau MD.

Figure 3.16 Reprinted with permission from Elsevier from Passerieux E., Rossignol R., Chopard A. et al. (2006) Structural organization of the perimysium in bovine skeletal muscle: Junctional plates and associated intracellular subdomains. *Journal of Structural Biology* 154 (2) 206–216.

Figure 3.18 Reproduced with kind permission from Christl Kiener Publishing.

Figure 3.19 Reproduced with kind permission from Thomas W. Myers and Lotus Publishing.

Figure 3.20 Reproduced with kind permission from Thomas W. Myers and Lotus Publishing.

Figure 3.21 Reproduced with kind permission from Thomas W. Myers and Lotus Publishing.

Figure 3.22 Reproduced with kind permission from Thomas W. Myers and Lotus Publishing.

Figure 3.23 Reproduced with kind permission from Thomas W. Myers and Lotus Publishing.

Figure 3.24 Reproduced with kind permission from Thomas W. Myers and Lotus Publishing.

Figure 3.25 Reproduced with kind permission from Thomas W. Myers and Lotus Publishing.

Figure 3.26 Reproduced with kind permission from Thomas W. Myers.

Figure 3.27 Adapted with kind permission from Jaap van der Wal.

Figure 3.28 Reproduced with permission from John Wiley & Sons. From Willard F. H., Vleeming A., Schuenke M. D., Danneels L., Schleip R. (2012) The thoracolumbar fascia: anatomy, function and clinical considerations. *Journal of Anatomy.* December; 221 (6) 507–536.

Figure 3.29 Adapted with permission from Handspring Publishing. From Luchau T. (2016) *Advanced Myofascial Techniques: Neck, Head, Spine and Ribs, Volume 2.* Edinburgh, UK: Handspring Publishing.

Figure 3.30 Image courtesy of Carla Stecco.

Figure 3.31 Photo by Lauri Nemetz. Reproduced with

permission from the Fascial Net Plastination Project, www.fasciaresearchsociety.org/plastination.

Figure 3.32 Reproduced with permission from the Fascial Net Plastination Project, www.fasciaresearchsociety.org/plastination.

Figure 3.33 Photo by Rachelle Clauson. Reproduced with permission from the Fascial Net Plastination Project, www.fasciaresearchsociety.org/plastination.

Figure 3.34 Photo by Stefan Westerback. Reproduced with permission from the Fascial Net Plastination Project, www.fasciaresearchsociety.org/plastination.

Figure 3.35 Photo by author. Reproduced with permission from the Fascial Net Plastination Project, www.fasciaresearchsociety.org/plastination.

Figure 3.36 Reproduced with permission from the Fascial Net Plastination Project, www.fasciaresearchsociety.org/plastination.

Figure 3.37 FR:EIA (Fascia Revealed: Educating Interconnected Anatomy) is the world's first 3-D human fascia plastinate.

It was created at Dr. Gunther von Hagens' Plastinarium in Guben Germany, by his BODY WORLDS team in collaboration with the Fascia Research Society. © www.BODYWORLDS.com/FR:EIA.

Figure 3.38 Reprinted with permission from Elsevier. From Scali F., Pontell M. E., Enix D. E., and Marshall E. (2013) Histological analysis of the rectus capitis posterior major's myodural bridge. *The Spine Journal.* May; 13 (5) 558–563.

Figure 3.39 Reprinted with permission from Elsevier. From Scali F., Pontell M. E., Enix D. E., and Marshall E. (2013) Histological analysis of the rectus capitis posterior major's myodural bridge. *The Spine Journal.* May; 13 (5) 558–563.

Figure 4.1 Reproduced with permission from Elsevier. From Tesarz J., Hoheisel U., Wiedenhöfer B., and Mense S. (2011) Sensory innervation of the thoracolumbar fascia in rats and humans. *Neuroscience.* October; 194, 302–308.

Figure 5.1 (B) Reproduced with kind permission from Maiken Nedergaard.

Figure 5.2 Reproduced with kind permission from Maiken Nedergaard.

Figure 5.3 Reproduced with kind permission from Tom Deerinck.

Figure 5.4 Image reproduced with kind permission from R. Douglas Fields and Hiroaki Wake, NIH.

Figure 5.6 Reproduced with kind permission from Jeff Johnson, Hybrid Medical Animations.

Figure 5.7 Photograph by D. Fawcett. Reproduced with kind permission from Science Source.

Figure 6.2 Photo by Nicole Trombley and Rachelle Clauson. Courtesy of AnatomySCAPES.com.

Figure 6.3 Modified with permission from Stecco L. and Stecco C. (2013) *Fascial Manipulation for Internal Dysfunctions.* Padova, Italy: Piccin Nuova Libraria S.p.A.

Figure 6.5 Image provided by Dr. Doris A. Taylor, Texas Heart Institute, Houston.

Figure 6.6 Reprinted with permission from John Wiley & Sons. From Ohtani O. and Ohtani Y. (2008) Lymph circulation in the liver. *The Anatomical Record: Advances in Integrative Anatomy and Evolutionary Biology.* June; 291 (6) 643–652.

Figure 7.7 Reproduced with permission from Christopher Gordon.

Figure 7.8 Reproduced with permission from Christopher Gordon.

Figure 7.9 Licensed by BioMed Central Ltd. From Langevin H. M., Fox J. R., Koptiuch C. et al. (2011) Reduced thoracolumbar fascia shear strain in human chronic low back pain. *BMC Musculoskeletal Disorder.* September; 12, 203 (2011). Open Access. Distributed under the terms of the Creative Commons Attribution License (http://creativecommons.org/licenses/by/2.0).

Figure 7.10 Reproduced with kind permission from Dr. Wolfgang Bauermeister.

Figure 8.1 Illustration adapted with permission from fascialnet.com.

Figure 8.2 Reprinted with permission from Elsevier. From Meltzer K. R., Cao T. V., Schad J. F. et al. (2010) In vitro modeling of repetitive motion injury and myofascial release. *Journal of Bodywork and Movement Therapies.* April; 14 (2) 162–171.

Figure 8.3 Reprinted with permission from John Wiley & Sons. From Langevin H. M., Churchill D. L., Wu J., et al. (2002) Evidence of connective tissue involvement in acupuncture. *FASEB Journal.* June; 16 (8) 872–874.

Figure 8.4 Reproduced with permission from Handspring Publishing. From Chaitow L. (ed.) (2014) *Fascial Dysfunction: Manual Therapy Approaches.* Edinburgh, UK: Handspring Publishing.

INDEX

Note: Bold page numbers refer to tables and italic page numbers refers to figures.

'I love the way David tells his story by first relating the facts and theories we all need for such a complex subject as fascia. Yet he covers extensive but essential material in a way that leaves you refreshingly in a state of wonderment instead of exhaustion. From there he departs from other authors by weaving in his own perspectives and unique experiences with fascia: as an experienced clinician; as a videographer of anything fascia; and as a genuinely thoughtful, feeling person who cares deeply about what he writes. I thoroughly enjoyed it and so will you.'

Chris Frederick, PT, Co-Director Stretch to Win Institute, Creators of Fascial Stretch Therapy™ www.StretchToWin.com

'I've had to translate the chapters of most fascia books for my clients and students – until now. Thank you David, for simplifying this complex subject and doing it in the most entertaining of ways. Fascia fundamentals at its absolute best!'

PJ O'Clair, Master Instructor Trainer at Merrithew, Senior Master Instructor TRX™, Owner of ClubXcel and Northeast Pilates

'David has done the miraculous! He's written a book on fascia that's a real page-turner. This entertaining and educating book illuminates fascia's meaning in your body and in life. David deftly navigates scientific breakthroughs with a rock and roll sensibility that will capture the imagination of movement educators, clinicians, manual therapists and anatomy geeks.'

Jill Miller, author of *'The Roll Model, A Step by Step Guide to Erase Pain, Improve Mobility and Live Better in Your Body'*

'Sensitively written with an admirable understanding of fascia's clinical importance and complex functions, this important book strips away myth, and provides clarity.'

Leon Chaitow ND DO, Honorary Fellow, University of Westminster, London, Editor-in-Chief, *Journal of Bodywork & Movement Therapies*

'I found Lesondak's writing style to be rich, insightful and engaging. I highly recommend his book as a must-have for any fascia library.'

Eric Franklin www.franklinmethod.com

'For every one interested in getting a better overview of the workings of fascia, this book will become your road map'.

Prof. Dr. Andry Vleeming, Program Chairman, World Congress Lumbopelvic Pain, Medical Osteopathic College of the University of New England, Maine USA, Department of Rehabilitation Sciences and Physiotherapy, Faculty of Medicine and Health Sciences, Ghent University